*I'm*possible

*My personal journey of living with
Ulcerative Colitis*

Heather B. Jacobs

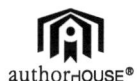

AuthorHouse™
1663 Liberty Drive
Bloomington, IN 47403
www.authorhouse.com
Phone: 1-800-839-8640

© 2014 Heather B. Jacobs. All rights reserved.

No part of this book may be reproduced, stored in a retrieval system, or transmitted by any means without the written permission of the author.

Published by AuthorHouse 5/12/2014

ISBN: 978-1-4969-0535-2 (sc)
ISBN: 978-1-4969-0534-5 (hc)
ISBN: 978-1-4969-0533-8 (e)

Library of Congress Control Number: 2014906952

Any people depicted in stock imagery provided by Thinkstock are models, and such images are being used for illustrative purposes only.
Certain stock imagery © Thinkstock.

Because of the dynamic nature of the Internet, any web addresses or links contained in this book may have changed since publication and may no longer be valid. The views expressed in this work are solely those of the author and do not necessarily reflect the views of the publisher, and the publisher hereby disclaims any responsibility for them.

This book is dedicated to strength, hope and resilience; wherever these may be found. And to my family for helping to instill each of these in me and for supporting me on my journey in discovering that I'm Possible.

Acknowledgements

I would like to thank my family for standing by me through every hard time that the last few years have brought to me. My mom and papa for making this journey possible and helping me create this story. My sister, Merel, for always believing in me - even when it was not easy. A very special thank you to Jeff Grabow for never giving up on me. Allison Hopkins for getting me started with this book and for her editing services. Sherry Moore for reading my manuscript and providing feedback. Lastly, I want to acknowledge all the doctors who did their best to help me, even if their help was not successful.

Message To Myself

People living with chronic disease must have an open mind because the disease and the body are always changing.

Even though it is hard at times and sometimes it seems easiest just to give up, the moment you give up nothing can help you.

Even though it is frustrating, sometimes you just have to scream and cry and let it out and then get back to caring for your body. As soon as you stop getting back up; you have been defeated.

As soon as you give up, you go from being possible to impossible.

Don't worry about being different or eating funny foods, because "Those who mind don't matter, and those who matter don't mind" (Dr. Seuss)

Nobody can truly understand what you are going through but people truly do care. truly do care. Even though only you can truly understand you cannot push people away because whether you realize it or not, they want to be there for you.

Find someone you trust to be there to hold your hand and wipe your tears; you don't have to fight alone.

Be able to laugh at yourself, believe in yourself and be confident that you will win this battle.

Don't stop living life the way you always planned to or the way you want to. The diagnosis is simply just a roadblock that will make your achievements that much more rewarding. Your disease may be the reason you cannot do some things but never let it be the excuse for doing nothing. True, it may make a lot of things more difficult, but not impossible.

My challenge is not impossible; because I'm possible.

My Life Changed Over Night June 10, 2010

I can't remember being so uncomfortable ever in my life: this hard bed, these thin sheets, and worst of all the blue walls and plexi-glass window. These pajamas they are making me wear have a huge opening in the back, and they think they make up for that by giving me a nice pair of itchy pants. It's all so unfamiliar to me. I long for my big comfy comforter and my pink walls, my flannel jammies and my own home.

My life changed last night and will never be the same. It all began with my graduation night. I graduated 8th grade from the Catholic school I had attended since kindergarten. Both of my grand moms were in town for that big night. It was an emotional one for me. My last year at school was a stressful year with lots of drama with both the teachers and the other students. I'm happy to be done, but also already a little nervous about starting high school. I will be moving up to a small town in the mountains in a few weeks and will start a new life there. My family had bought some land there a few years ago to build a vacation cabin, which then became a dream house, which will soon be our home. I'm sad to leave my friends and the people I've known all my life, but I know that I will love my new home and moving will be a good experience.

So how did I end up in this hospital bed? Well, when my graduation ceremony was finally over, my mom, dad, little sister, my grand moms and I were going to celebrate with dinner at my favorite Italian restaurant. Everyone was excited! But, in the car on the way there I began to complain of stomach pain. I thought it was nothing; that I was just hungry, so we continued onward to dinner. All was great, food was delicious and everyone had a good time. We all went off to bed, exhausted after a long day and the next morning headed up to our mountain house. That is when the trouble started. Without any warning, I started having more and more stomach pain and bleeding. I was freaking out!! My mom took me straight to the doctor. They ordered some tests, took my blood and some poop and sent us home.

Over the next two days, I just got worse. My mom called the doctor and she said the lab results weren't back yet. At about 2AM on the third day, I woke up, sick as a dog. I spent an hour in the bathroom and then passed out - Stone cold on the bathroom floor. My mom bundled me up and headed for the emergency room…and so the journey began.

My mom and I sat in the cold emergency room for at least 2 hours with nothing to show, but a wristband. In severe pain I sat curled in a ball in a waiting room chair. I watched person after person go in to see the doctor before me. Some with broken arms, some just wanted drugs, and others you could see were in pain. There was one man I remember distinctly. He was old, about 85, and was with a younger woman, his daughter I imagine. They too had been waiting for hours and began to get fed-up. The woman went over to the ER nurse and started yelling at her. She was saying that the man was in severe pain and if someone didn't help him now he would die right there. We looked over at the man who was sitting in a plastic blue chair like the rest of us, but he seemed quite content. He didn't appear to be in great pain nor did he appear to be dying. This frustrated me, because I knew that I needed help immediately, but I waited as multiple over-reacting phonies passed through the doctor's doors. I wondered how there could be so many people in the ER at 4 in the morning! My mom held me in her arms until finally my name was called, "Heather Jacobs".

Must have slept another couple of hours in the ER, because the next thing I remember was being in a wheelchair to be taken by ambulance to another hospital. I'm kind of mad about not being allowed to walk myself. It's not like I'm some kind of mental patient or a big flight risk! The wheelchair was probably a good idea though, since I kept passing out. That was better than being strapped onto a gurney in the ambulance. Only good thing was that one of the paramedics that lifted me into the ambulance was totally cute. Too bad I looked like crap.

I don't have my own room. I am in ICU and I am sharing with two other children. One is a baby, a few months old, I would guess. She has lots of IVs and sleeps, lifelessly. Then, there is the boy. He is about 4 years old and very confused. He doesn't understand why he is here and is insistently asking questions that can't be answered, like, "when are we going home?" There are constantly nurses, doctors and people coming into my curtain room. The worst visitor was the priest. He asked *if I needed to give confession before he went home for the night!* He acted like I was going to die. Am I going to die?

Just a few hours ago my nurse came in to give me a new IV. This time it's a 20 gauge, whatever that means. The first IV didn't hurt that bad, just a pinch, but this one, oh man! She poked my arm and instantly blood shot at least a foot into the air and covered my nice thin sheets. I already didn't like her, and then she said, "Oops, sorry about that, you have small veins." Yesterday, I had big easy veins and today they are small? I'm confused. I wonder what the next one will be like? Ouch…

"Welcome To Hell. We Have Pee-Water." June 11, 2010

Last night was a hard night for me. Not only because of the pain and the constant trips to my personal toilet, but because of what I heard. The baby across the way (the one that is only a few months) didn't make it through the night. I was lying in my bed, partially asleep, when I heard her monitor sound out. Her lifeline had gone flat and the alarm sounded. Nurses came running from every direction; doing everything they could to resuscitate her. But nothing could be done. When they turned off her machine, the cries from her father, who had never left her side, broke my heart. He had lost his baby.

I know that this memory will never leave me, because it truly broke my heart. Words cannot describe the feelings this memory left behind.

I don't have my own bathroom, well I guess in a sense I do. It's portable. A small plastic toilet that they wheel into my room whenever I have to go is what I have to call my porcelain throne. I have to have some tests done, which means I have to drink some disgusting stuff that tastes like pee-water. The test is a Meckel's Exam to see if I was born with a little pouch of stomach growing into my intestine. Therefore, I am forcing down this pee-water so the doctor can image my tummy.

Seems like I was under that metal pan for hours, but it was only half an hour of no movement whatsoever. Just the sound of clunks like the two-ton chunk of metal suspended from the ceiling was going to come crashing down and smash me flat onto the cold, hard table.

+++++++++

Okay, so I don't have Meckel's Diverticulum. That's good, but now it just means more tests...

Now I am moving on to an Endoscopy and a Colonoscopy. With the Endoscopy they are going to put a tube down my throat to see into my stomach and intestines. With the Colonoscopy, they are going to go the other direction...up my butt.

It might be nice to get out of this curtained room for a little while. Last night, around 1:00AM, the sheriff and a bunch of other people came into the curtain room to talk to the doctors about a six-year old boy who had just come in. Apparently, he fell down the stairs at home; they think his mom pushed him… There was a lot of yelling and they were only about 3 feet and a curtain away. The boy was bleeding, the father was crying and the mother was very upset at the police. It was being threatened that CPS was going to be called…I wonder if they were.

On the other side of me is a child who looks like a man, but he is in a crib. He screams a scream that doesn't sound like speaking. It sounds like the groan of a walrus in severe pain. And I know that he must be suffering, but I don't know what of.

I hate it here. Everywhere I look there is pain, and suffering and fear of the unknown.

I am scared and it doesn't help that I have to jump on the plastic toilet next to my bed every half hour.

Meeting Doctor Asshole, MD *June 11, 2010*

Well now I have no idea where I am. Last thing I remember I was in the pre-op area with a Russian lady putting sleep drugs into the IV in my arm. Shortly after that, the T.V. shot a mile away and then came super close to my face. Lights Out!

So now I am in a private, sterile room. No more curtain room, but still super thin sheets. At least I have my own bathroom and a shower.

Still a little loopy when my grand mom came in. She was a little confused about what was going on and freaked out just a tad. My sister and my dad were with her. My sister, Merel, brought me knitting supplies; to have something to do all day and my dad brought a bag of clean underwear.

My next visitors were the doctors. With them was the one I like to call "Dr. Asshole, MD." He was a real prick! Right away he started telling me that he does lots of surgeries and takes out lots of colons. "Sometimes kids get new ones, but not always", he said. "The kids that don't get a new colon get a colostomy bag." Basically, this is a bag attached to the outside of their stomach that their poop goes into. That's disgusting! ... No way!

There is a whiteboard in my room. It is attached to my bathroom door so we can record how much and how often I poop. It was a lot and mostly blood. So I decided to use the whiteboard as a tribute to Dr. Asshole MD. I wrote his 'name' all over it!! Then, unfortunately, the medical students came in to ask the same questions again, "Have I been drinking lake water? Had we travelled out of the country? Had I been drinking anything to poison myself?" No, no, no. That's when my mom blew a gasket and told them all to get out! It was a little bit embarrassing.

+++++++++

The nurses keep coming in to get my 'stool samples'. I actually have to poop into a bucket in the toilet, and then my mom has to measure how much and then call the nurses. It smells yucky. Mostly blood, so it doesn't smell like poop.... Worse!

Now, the nurses are wearing gloves, and gowns and masks since apparently I have been put into 'isolation' because I am now contagious. That's new. The nurses look like those guys on Monster's Inc. who shower down the monsters after they touch a kid! Boy, that makes me feel super special.

Sneaking Out Of Isolation   *June 12, 2010*

I'm allowed to eat today. I was excited until I saw the menu. Not a lot of choices on a "Low-residue diet". It seemed like Mac-n-cheese would be a good choice, but they managed to make it disgusting. I passed it around to my family so everyone could taste how bad it was. It literally tasted like someone had thrown-up on a bowl of noodles!! My dad refused to taste it. The sight alone was enough for him. There was a bowl of jello… there was always a bowl of jello…that was good.

So now…I am hungry.

I am so glad mom got some white bread from the cafeteria. It's crazy that we snuck out of isolation to eat some bread. Mom thought a "picnic" with some fresh air would be nice, so we walked to the courtyard on our floor. It was kind of tricky walking with my IV pole and hospital gown, but I did it. The nurses saw me walking out and even said hello. Then, just as I was finishing my bread and butter, we got busted!

One of the nurses came out and yelled at me because I was an "isolation patient and could be infecting all of the others". The nurse this morning obviously didn't get the memo because she came in without the Monster's Inc. sterile-team costume and suggested that some fresh air would be nice today.

So…we walked back to our room.

On the way I saw a boy in a wheelchair. He was bald, and his family surrounded him, all crying hysterically. I did not know what was going on until I overheard them speaking. "It is going to be okay, you will be with Jesus soon".
They were saying goodbye…

There are no words to express the feeling that comes over someone when they witness something like that. A child, with his whole life still ahead of him, had to say goodbye, too soon.

This is when I realized that others had it worse… and that I was going to be okay. I had to be.

+++++++++

It is kind of late now, but the nurse just took my IV out and said I could have my first shower. Having an IV pulled – slowly pulled- out of your vein is definitely something you can feel. A shower is also something you can feel. And boy did that feel good!

Beep Beep Beeeeeeep......   *June 13, 2010*

Today was a long day... My mom and I have been forced to take up knitting. I have been released from isolation and moved to a new room— which should be a good thing – but my new nurses freaked out as soon as I fell asleep. My heart rate goes too low. That led to a full EKG to basically inform everyone that since I am an athlete my heart rate runs low.

Papa and sissy visited. They decided to mix things up a bit and ride their bikes to the hospital.

Basically today was spent knitting and visiting. After knitting we enjoyed a gourmet dinner consisting of rubber salmon, cold rice and frozen peas. All I can say is thank God for the jello.

M...R...I...

June 14, 2010

Sissy brought me a teddy bear last night that she won at the amusement park. My dad brought me more clean underwear. Thanks Papa! I slept with that teddy bear all night. He is kind of ugly... in a cute sort of way. I'm not really sure if it is a dog or a bear. The head, at least twice as big as the body, has plastic eyes and a big smile. My teddy dog is the same pale blue color as the sheets.

+++++++++

Today is the day I get sent into the magnetic tube. Yippee! MRI day... Too bad my teddy dog can't go with me. He's gone. He got folded up in the sheets and taken away. I went to the bathroom for two minutes and the nurse changed the sheets with my teddy dog in them. If only he had been a different color.

No one told me I was going to be forced to drink 3 liters of Barium – worse than the Pee Water. Barium resembles ground up, pureed puke and tastes about the same. After handing me three bottles of this nasty stuff, the nurse informed me that I had 15 minutes to finish it all. Fifteen minutes seems like a long time, but not when you are on the edge of puking up every sip. Then it seems like a lifetime. At first, I took my time, but then was told I would lose my time slot for the test if I didn't finish it all, so I downed the last bottle in 5 minutes... Take that!

To make matters worse, I was drinking Barium when I met the child therapist. Short, wavy brown hair and a squeaky voice. She said she was here for me if I needed to talk or wanted to be comforted during this tough time. She also said she was available for my parents and family because this would be a tough time for them too. I don't think I will be calling her any time soon. If anything, she seems like she would just make matters worse. Her voice drove me crazy, and she kept touching my arm when she talked - little did she know that blood had just shot out of it and it hurt! She was supposed to help me feel calm while I had to drink three bottles of barium in 15 minutes.... Not helping! She then felt the need to inform me that *"I might feel like I am suffocating... then I might need to throw-up while strapped to the table... Which could then cause me to suffocate..."* She also let me know that *"the noise can be deafening..."* Then she reassured me with some goggles *"so you can watch Little Mermaid."* Yeah... while you slide me into this magnetic tomb that I can't escape from, I will remember how much I love Little Mermaid.

I guess the mean Barium Nurse wasn't so bad after all. After my horrifying experience inside the loudest, coldest cylinder imaginable I was greeted by a stuffed Panda bear from the gift shop, seated on my wheelchair. My mom had told the nurse about my missing teddy dog while I was in the MRI, so the nurse got me the panda.

Home At Last!!!   *June 14, 2010*

It is late and I am exhausted, but I'm home. It's just my mom and me. Merel and Papa have gone up to our new house in the mountains because we are in the process of moving. We built a house up there about two years ago and have decided to make that house our home. My sister will be starting 6th grade at a whole new school and I, a freshman in high school.

I have Ulcerative Colitis. The doctors told us it is an autoimmune disease that I will have the rest of my life. Basically, my body is attacking my own colon and leaving big, bleeding ulcers behind. They told me to get used to life with a chronic disease, because now it will forever be a part of my life…

My mom and I looked it up on the Internet, to find out exactly what it is that I have. What I learned is that:

> *Ulcerative Colitis is an inflammatory disease that is most commonly treated with special anti-inflammatory and/or immune blocking drugs. It is a disease that affects about 250,000-500,000 Americans. The cause of Ulcerative Colitis is still unknown but there are several theories as to why it appears and how to treat it. The leading theory is that an over-reaction of the immune system causes the body to attack the lining of the colon. But there are other theories about food sensitivities, bacterial imbalances and viruses. The symptoms include severe abdominal pain, frequent bowel movements and/or diarrhea with blood in the poop, joint pain, hemorrhoids, chronic fatigue and anemia. Conventional medical treatments are prescription medications including oral amino salicylates and mesalamines, which are aspirin-like compounds, and steroids. If these don't work, then immune-blocking medications may be prescribed or surgical removal of part or all of the colon may be necessary.*

Wow! That is heavy. Tonight, when I lay in bed I noticed something new. I have lost a lot of weight over the last couple of days. Every bone in my hips and rib cage are protruding. I look like a skeleton.

Treatment Plan   June 15, 2010

Today I woke up in my own bed in our own house. It's a good feeling. But, I guess it is not really home anymore. I'm sad that Papa and sissy have already moved up to our new house. I can't believe this is happening...

Although the rush to the toilet every morning still hasn't changed, my symptoms have decreased dramatically - down from about 20 bloody discharges a day to about 9. That's progress. And I get to eat. It is supposed to be "low residue" which means white bread, rice, applesauce, chicken and pears. At least it's not hospital food.

The doctors sent me home with a truck lode of pills. Pills to treat the Ulcerative Colitis, pills to treat the problems caused by the other pills, and pills to kill the parasites in my gut. Yep, I have parasites. "Blastocystis Hominis" which is apparently a bug we all have in our guts, but mine decided to overproduce. So, my list of pills includes:

<u>Sulfasalazine</u> – (used to stop the inflammation in Ulcerative Colitis) comes with a long list of scary side effects

> *Fever*
> *Sore throat*
> *Appearance of a rash*
> *Easy bruising*
> *Pain when urinating*
> *Appearance of an entire tablet in bowel movement*
> *Ringing in ears*
> *White patches in mouth or on lips*
> *Dizziness*
> *Sensitive to sun exposure*

WHAT??? It is the first week of summer vacation, we have a neighborhood pool at our new house, and I am going to be sensitive to sun exposure? I hate this.

<u>Mesalamine Suppositories</u> (AKA: Butt Rockets – basically the same as sulfasalazine but NOT taken by mouth) These are not fun to take... They

are like little bullets that I have to stick up my butt so that the medicine can get to the lower parts of my colon; quickly.

Folic Acid Supplements – (since Sulfasalazine depletes folic acid)

Metronidazole (Flagyl) – (to kill the parasite).

So many pills, but I'm just happy to be out of the hospital, away from Dr. Asshole, MD and on the way to being healthy again!

Glass, Staples And Nails

June 25, 2010

Up early and on the road. We are driving back to the hospital. Today is the day of my first follow-up appointment with my GI doctors. At least I won't have to see Dr. Asshole MD, instead it's the Gastroenterologist and his fellow. I'm nervous.

+++++++++

So, my appointment went pretty well. The medications appear to be working and the game plan is to stay on the Sulfasalazine at least until I get through the stress of my first year of high school. Then, my doctors re-evaluate and decide which medication to put me on for the rest of my life.

Pills forever can't be that bad. At least it's better than hospital gowns and bedpans!

One thing that did happen at the appointment that annoyed me just a tad was when my mommy brought up my 'low residue diet'. She went on to ask if I had to continue eating that way. Then my Gastroenterologist so kindly stated that "No, I did not need to continue the diet, but unfortunately I could no longer eat glass, staples and nails, because there are holes in my colon."

That comment may seem like a joke, but nobody should joke about holes in their intestines with someone who was just discharged from the week of hell that would change their life forever.

And that someone is Me.

Doing Okay, But Not Great   *July 4, 2010*

It's the fourth of July! The lake is the place to be. There are tons of people packed into its vicinities to celebrate our Nation's Birthday, and we are here to do just that! A bunch of our ski buddies from the race team are meeting us soon for a BBQ and party at the lake. Today is going to be fun.

+++++++++

It's late now and I'm back home in bed. Today was great. Everyone had so much fun at the lake. Only one thing could have made the day even better: less pain. Ever since I was discharged I have this random pain in my tummy, it comes and goes but when it comes it is so bad it makes me want to cry. To add to the pain, my tummy talks. It roars so loud that people probably think I haven't eaten in weeks. But it doesn't roar because I'm hungry, it roars because my body is angry; and it has a lot to say. The pain was hard to deal with at the lake because all I wanted to do was have some carefree fun, but every once in a while that pain would come along to remind me that fun was easy to find but who knew how long it would be until that fun could be carefree again.

Sunshine And Sunscreen   August 1, 2010

Summer in the mountains is way more fun than summer in the city. We have the lakes, the pool, the hiking and the biking – so much to do. I have also started going to summer workouts for volleyball at my new high school. Already meeting people and making new friends! I am a little bit nervous for high school but still pretty excited. The biggest bummer this summer is my mom chasing me with the sunscreen. Unfortunately, I didn't know I had to sunscreen my eyes, so I burned my eyeballs – ouch! When the doctors started me on Sulfasalazine they failed to mention that even my eyes would be sensitive to the sun.

We have these camping beds and a great big porch, 22 feet off the ground. So, I have been sleeping outside almost every night. There is a meteor shower in a couple of days. Plan is to wake up at 4:00 in the morning to watch! Shouldn't be too hard for me since I seem to be up most the night thinking. Seems funny that I'm having so much fun but I still feel sad.

Feeling Sad   *August 9, 2010*

Today is another follow-up appointment with the GI specialists.

My mommy and I left early this morning because we had to drop off stool samples at the clinic laboratory. We had never been to this clinic before and they had told us just to collect MY "specimen" in a tupperware to bring to the clinic… kinda strange. Then they would transfer it into the necessary vials for testing. Collecting my "sample" that morning was quite interesting. I had never tried to 'collect' without the little thing that goes in the potty to catch my doodie. So… mommy and I made our own! It was a tupperware taped into a paper plate. It worked! Good news is that it was easy to catch because my poop is good and there is no blood…

I mentioned to the doctors that I was feeling kind of sad. It seemed to me that maybe the medicine was making me feel that way because normally I am "Happy Heather" all the time. Well, most of the time. The doctors didn't agree with me. They said that was impossible. They told me that there are some stresses naturally associated with starting high school. Then, once again they felt the need to hit a soft spot and remind me that I was in a new town and didn't have friends yet. So, it's sulfa 'til December. We planned to follow-up in December to re-assess my medications.

Something Is Wrong   *August 11, 2010*

School is starting in a few days and I'm nervous. I'm in a new town with new people and a place where I know no one... The only faces that are familiar are those from my volleyball team that I have been practicing with all summer, but they already know each other from grade school.

I've been thinking about death a lot lately...

I'm not really sure what brought on all this thinking, but I can't help myself. Every time I watch a movie and someone dies I can't control the tears. I can't watch the news because any time I do, I have a panic attack. And suicide is a topic I cannot even bear to hear about.

I don't know were all of this has come from but it is starting to scare me. For the last few days I have cried myself to sleep and every time I close my eyes I see horrible things: things that just the thought of gives me the chills.

When I was in middle school we had this lecture about teen bullying and suicide. The teacher told a story about a boy who was cyber bullied by some kids at school and eventually committed suicide by hanging himself in the shower. The presentation included a slide show image of the shower where the boy died. That image did not affect all the students the way it did me. That picture of the dark shower with the transparent curtain is forever embedded in my brain, and when I close my eyes at night, I see that shower. I can't help but think of the boy and why he did what he did. I think about how hard life must have been for him, but wonder why he would take his own life. This used to baffle me; I could never imagine suicide. But now this idea has become less foreign to me.

+++++++++

Today, the thoughts got out of control.

Any time I saw a rope, I thought to hang myself. If there was a knife on the counter I thought of all the horrible things that could have been done with that knife. I couldn't take a shower without breaking down in tears and if I was left alone for more than a few seconds I lost control of my thoughts and did not know were I was. Then, seconds later I would be able to see myself, as a kind of out-of-body experience, curled in a ball, shaking and crying.

I don't know what is going on.

I came to the conclusion today that it was time to tell someone about this. But how? It's not exactly an easy conversation to bring up…

My mom was folding laundry when I walked in and asked, "Why do people kill themselves?"

Instantly she knew something was wrong, I could tell. She must have been thinking, *"What is happening to my daughter? Happy Heather is asking questions about suicide?"*

She answered that suicide was a horribly sad thing, but some people feel that they have too much pain to continue living. My questions continued in asking if people my age kill themselves a lot.

I broke down crying.

I told her everything I had been experiencing and eventually found myself lying on the floor, hysterical. I told her that I don't want to kill myself or hurt myself in any way but I keep thinking about it even though I don't want to be.

She is scared, I am scared and I don't know where all of this is coming from… this isn't me.

Something is wrong.

It Must Be The Sulfasalazine... August 13, 2010

These bad thoughts aren't getting any better; they just get worse and worse and worse. It must be the medicine. That is all that has changed. Before I got sick I was Happy Heather, then as soon as my disease became a part of my life, Happy Heather went away... where did she go?

My mom and I had a long talk about whether this medicine could possibly cause all of these thoughts. The doctors never mentioned ANYTHING about suicidal ideations when they gave me the list of side effects.

We called the doctor and told them about what we had been noticing and wondered if it had to do with the medicine.

They answered positively that it was impossible that the medicine had anything to do with this and that I was simply depressed.

Depressed from the trauma of the hospital, the realization that my life would never be the same, the horrible things that I saw in the ICU, the pain and sadness I had experienced, and the difficulty of a chronic illness. Therefore, I was depressed and they informed me that this was part of what I would have to overcome. They also said that any kid who has to start high school in a new town is certain to have anxiety and depression. It was not because of the medication, it was because I am a teenager with a chronic illness.

Cutest Boy In School   August 18, 2010

Today is that day…. First day of school! I'm nervous.

+++++++++

So, it went great!

School was awesome. I had nothing to be worried about. When the bell rang for lunch, I wandered around aimlessly for only a minute or two until a few of the girls from volleyball invited me to eat with them. We ate lunch together and all had a great time telling stories about our classes and the people we had met. My teachers are all much nicer than I had expected and I like most of my classes, but I <u>really</u> like my math class…

There is this boy.

When I sat down in class today I scanned the room for anyone from my volleyball team. There were two girls and I happened to sit fairly close to both of them. But, across the room I caught eyes with the cutest boy in school. All class we looked up at each other and as soon as we caught eyes we both quickly looked away, and then instantly looked up to stare at each other again. I learned nothing that period… He is so cute!

After class when everyone jumped up at the sound of the bell and headed for the door, the cute boy approached me and stuck out his hand. His deep voice caught me off guard and I didn't know what to do… HE WAS TALKING TO ME!
Taking my hand firmly into his, he introduced himself and shot me a smile. Jeff Grabow… That's a name I won't forget.

YIPPIE!!!
Maybe High School won't be so bad after all…

Happy Birthday To Me! August 27, 2010

It's been a long day. My birthday is supposed to be a special day where everything goes my way and it's all about smiles and the birthday girl, but today was not that day.

I woke up to see party streamers that my parents have always hung the night before my birthday for me to wake up to on my special day. But only being able to enjoy them for a matter of seconds, I had to run to the bathroom.

Bloody Diarrhea at least 4 times before school is not how I wanted to spend my birthday.

I shouldn't have expected anything different, this is how I wake up most mornings lately, but for some reason I hoped that my birthday would be different.

I will have to literally run to the bathroom, with about 30 seconds tops before I lose control and ruin my Victoria's Secret undies. Thankfully my undies were safe today!

At school I felt different; just not myself. Not to mention it was about 100 degrees outside. When I look around I wonder what everyone's story is. The gothic boy who sits in the corner with his hair over his eyes, all alone, why? The football jock who acts like he doesn't have a care in the world, does he? The girls who travel in packs and whisper to each other, what are they saying? Do the girls on my volleyball team really like me? Why is the short girl so mean to everyone if she just met us, who is she to judge? Why does the world work the way it does? Where do I fit in?

I was sad after school, but I shouldn't have been. I just cannot stop the sadness. I knew I would come home to a beautiful devil's food chocolate cake with fluffy vanilla frosting, sitting on the counter awaiting my arrival. When I walked in the door I was slightly more excited, especially when the thought of eating that wonderful cake crossed my mind. My cake was decorated with a smiley face that my mother had frosted by hand for her Happy Heather. I loved it but still didn't feel myself inside.

I feel like I am faking my happiness.

My birthday dinner was all eaten up and the array of incredible gifts from everyone in my family had been opened, so we headed down to our basement to watch my favorite movie of all time, "*27 Dresses*"!

When the movie had ended we all headed up for bed because unfortunately it is a school night. Yet, after being sung to and hugged by my family I burst into tears. It was hysterical crying and sadness about nothing at all. I then muttered under my tears that I was sad my dad hadn't played "Happy Birthday" on his saxophone for me like he always has. He quickly got his saxophone and was able to clear my tears with the sound of his incredibly loud version of the song.

But this was all just an excuse, I don't really know why I am so sad, but I am. I have no control over my feelings; it feels like there is a different person living in my body. I lay here in bed, covered in tears, just praying that I can be happy again soon… what a birthday it has been.

Flares — *August 30, 2010*

Right now I am taking three, 500 mg pills of Sulfasalazine daily. The doctors said I had a flare and that is to be expected sometimes. Apparently this disease is like a rollercoaster; the symptoms can come back and then go away at any time for various reasons. So, now my colitis is under control and my health is great, but my mental situation has not gotten any better.

I keep trying to tell the doctors that this medicine is making me crazy but nobody, except my mom will listen to me.

My Body Is Burning!

September 1, 2010

My skin feels tingly on my stomach, it itches like crazy and I just wish I could peel my skin off! The strange thing is that only the right half of my stomach is having these sensations, everything to the left of my belly button feels normal.

I have no idea why; maybe it's just a pulled muscle.

By around lunchtime today the tingling turned into severe burning, I couldn't turn to the side and a sit up seemed to be about the most painful thing imaginable.

I figured I just pulled a muscle and lathered myself with Aspercreme. The pain is increasing and all I want to do is sleep, so that is exactly what I plan to do. Hopefully it's gone by tomorrow, whatever it is...

It Wasn't A Pulled Muscle   *September 5, 2010*

My body has been itching and burning for a few days with me still thinking the least of it and trying to ignore the pain. After a while I figured it probably wasn't a pulled muscle and stopped applying Aspercreme. I hoped this was not another reaction to the medicine and that it would pass.

Until today…

My mom called the Advice Nurse at the Hospital and she suggested it was simply Poison Oak. So, I (as gently as possible) rubbed TechNu all over my stomach and back…which was one of the most painful things I have ever done.

The nurse had assured us that pairing that with Benadryl and a generic cortisone cream would make it feel better. She said I must be hypersensitive to Poison Oak.

It's SHINGLES!   September 6, 2010

The burning is now accompanied with nausea and a pounding headache. When I open my eyes everything seems blurry for a second or two and then sharpens up quickly. My skin is throbbing and has the most severe burning sensation I have ever experienced and now, there is a rash...

This is not just any rash.

My rash looks like un-popped zits or boils in a line across the right side of my stomach, waiting to burst and surrounded by red irritation. Even just wearing a shirt is excruciatingly painful. Mixed around the rash are small blister-looking spots and I have what appears to be scratch marks across my back...

The car ride to urgent care was not a very comfortable one. Having to lean forward so that my back would not touch the seat and squeezing the chair any time we hit a bump were the accommodations that had to be made due to the severe tenderness and pain that my body was in.

Urgent care identified my rash as a definite Shingles rash and was shocked to see someone of my age with Shingles. They told us that the previous nurse probably suggested that I simply had Poison Oak because she might not have even thought to assess me for shingles at my age. Usually Shingles is found in people over the age of 50!

I was prescribed Acyclovir and Prednisone. I just want to be healthy again!

No More Shingles! September 18, 2010

Last week, going to school with a shingles rash had been an interesting experience. I have one friend who is an avid hugger and she didn't completely understand that my body was on fire and that I really didn't want a hug. The first day I went to school with the rash she came up and (not thinking about it) I hugged her back, yet it only took a matter of seconds to realize that hugging was unbelievably painful.

I didn't tell anyone, because having a nasty, oozy rash down your side isn't exactly the best way to make friends, and I'm still trying to do that! So, I told "Little Miss Hugs a Lot" that I was really sore from working out and hugging made it hurt more. She bought it and nobody ever saw my rash.

I went the rest of the week just walking carefully, trying not to bump anything and carrying my bag away from my side.

Except, volleyball was an issue…. diving, serving, hitting… this all involves stretching out your abdomen… and mine had been on fire all week!

One day, I even had to tell the coach I wasn't feeling well and wanted to sit out of practice. He told me "I looked fine" and if I sat out I wouldn't play in the next game. I didn't know what to do. To everyone else I look normal, but nobody knows my situation…I pushed through practice, which was probably not the best idea but I couldn't face the shame of sitting out and having everyone think I was faking to get out of practice.

That night I couldn't sleep, because just laying in bed was painful, not to mention shifting in my sleep. Once I finally fell asleep, I was woken up by the pain… It was a long night!

+++++++++

But now, my shingles are cleared and that week of guarding my stomach like it was the Holy Grail is over, but my moods are a mess!

Sometimes I am happy and other times I feel like I am going to kill myself, literally.

It is an absolutely horrible feeling to not have any control of your thoughts. One minute my body decides that it is so happy and wants to laugh and giggle about everything and then next, all I want to do is hide under my blanket and cry.

I still wonder why others commit suicide and wonder if I ever would. My brain tells me that I should sometimes, but as a person I don't want to and never would. There are voices in my head…

It sounds crazy and I never thought it was real, but I honestly can hear voices telling me that I don't need to be here anymore and to just do it.

I cry because I am scared.

What is one supposed to do about this… am I crazy?

I don't want to die, I have so much to live for and I know that. Never once have I, in my right mind, ever wanted to hurt myself in any way… so then why are these voices here? I want them gone!

It has to be the medicine. I am convinced! But I can't just stop taking the Sulfasalazine. Even decreasing the dosage can be dangerous and cause my disease to return, so I am going to have to find another way to deal with whatever is going on in my head.

I don't want anyone to think I am crazy, I just wish they could understand. I don't want to scare my mom and have her think I'm suicidal, but telling her I'm hearing voices isn't exactly easy either…

Trick-or-Treat   October 30, 2010

Life has been pretty good lately. I do my best to push the bad thoughts aside and stay busy. School is great, I've made some good friends, volleyball is over now but I got the "Most Improved Player" award and the cutest boy in school is still looking at me!

Life is good. I've started meditating and trying to gain better control of my mind so that when a scary thought comes on I can try and push it away. My mom got me this music CD that is supposed to help the brain form positive thoughts. It doesn't always work, but it helps. I call it my "Magic Music" because whether or not it pushes the thoughts away it can make me fall asleep in a matter of minutes!

+++++++++

I got invited to go trick-or-treating with some friends tonight! Not having anything to wear for a costume my mom, sister and I went and got some funny matching top and bottom pajamas, my friends painted freckles on my face, braided my hair in two side braids and I carried around I stuffed dog! I was a little kid!

I might be a little old for trick-or-treating, but it's free candy and we had so much fun! There was this man who played the usual trick-or-treat chainsaw scare but he didn't do it quite right!

Usually someone will run around the neighborhood with a chainsaw that DOESN'T HAVE A CHAIN ON and try to scare all of the trick-or-treaters, but this man had the chain on his saw and he was getting really close to people! It was so terrifying that my friends and I took off at a full sprint and one girl even fell into a ditch, but we all just kept on running!

Another fun story from tonight was my friend's desperate need to pee! There was nowhere to pee since we were out wandering the neighborhoods in search of candy, but we came upon this one darkened house with a car out front. On Halloween, having the porch lights off is the universal sign for "no trick-or-treat" we figured that was the most private place we were going to find. The rest of the street was swarming with kids! So, my friend went behind the parked car, pulled her pants down and let it rip! Once she finished and was walking toward the rest of us the car lights turned on and the engine started.... There was someone inside!

I Love London But I Hate My Brain! November 17, 2010

I have only dreamed of going to London and Paris! Now it's Thanksgiving Break and I am finally here! This trip is something I have been looking forward to for so long!

The first few days have been great, sight seeing - Big Ben, London Castle, Parliament, Westminster Abbey, Trafalgar Square— and we took a boat down the River Thames. London is beautiful and all I had imagined! The way the city lights up at night is magnificent and the people are all so proper. When the sun goes down, watching the London Eye spin with an array of brilliant colors across the water is a beautiful sight!

The food is kind of bland, but I love the big English Breakfast: toast, eggs, baked beans, boiled tomato and lots of ketchup.

Something funny happened today in Trafalgar Square:

> There is this beautiful fountain that my sister and I decided to jump in front of and take a picture mid air. We did this for a few minutes, trying to get a good picture and then noticed a crowd had formed around us. People were taking pictures and watching us jump! Like we were performers or something! We felt like celebrities and continued jumping! One older man even ran up to my papa and showed him the photo of us he had taken.

London is amazing! I just wish I could enjoy it more. The sad thoughts linger in the back of my mind wherever we are.

When we are touring around the city on a double decker bus I see myself jumping off of it, or when we took the boat along the river I imagined jumping in. When I look at Big Ben I see myself plummeting from the top and when I shower, I imagine a noose hanging from the showerhead.

It's driving me crazy!! I just want to be able to enjoy a fun family vacation without some voices in my head trying to kill me!

Welcome To Paris!   *November 19, 2010*

This morning we hopped on a train and took it from London, England to Paris, France; which in order to get between the two one must cross the English Channel. So, we did just that! Our train went <u>under water</u> beneath the Channel and brought us to Paris!

Paris is a land of beauty and poise, graced with The Louvre, Arc de Triomphe, The Champs-Élysées, Mont Marte, and the famous Eiffel Tower.

Our hotel room is incredible! We peer off our balcony with a direct view of the Eiffel Tower. Beautiful, strong and tall, the tower stood along the green lawns leading up to it. The smell of fresh baked bread and biscuits fills the air and our morning breakfast plate is stacked with custards, croissants, biscuits and other fresh baked goods. Delish!

+++++++++

We visited The Louvre today; the home of the Mona Lisa and a remarkable building in itself. The art and sculptures were awesome, and the building itself is really remarkable. For lunch we stopped at an eloquent little bakery where my sister and I bought two fresh baguettes; one for each of us. We took these baguettes to Tuileries Garden where we embarked on a laughter filled sword fight.

Today was such a fun day! Everything seems to be fine during the day. I am distracted with the fun of traveling this beautiful city all day, but when night falls my thoughts begin to wander.

Tonight, after a beautiful French dinner my family decided to take a walk through the streets of Paris in search of dessert! We came upon a corner crepe shop and each ordered up the crepe of our choice. Mine, being slathered with Nutela. I love French food!

Right now, as I lay here in my fluffy white bed with an array of pillows, I can't get the sad thoughts out of my head. There are demons in my mind. But, I am deciding tonight to stick to "Mind Over Matter" and keep myself focused on the wonderful day I had in this remarkable city and the fluffy pillows surrounding me.

Goodnight.

To A Good Day   *November 20, 2010*

Today was a good day!

We toured around Paris and enjoyed great food, a beautiful place and a wonderful vacation.

We toured the Arc de Triomphe and walked The Champs-Élysées. There was a festival set up along The Champs-Élysées where we bought souvenirs from local artists and vendors. We watched as an Army procession marched around the Arc and drank hot cocoa in a French café.

It was incredible!

For dessert we found a charming restaurant where we each ordered a large slice of our favorite cake; mine being a decadent chocolate slice, of course. Sitting on the patio, about 300 feet from the base of the Eiffel Tower, we watched as the tower flashed colors and lit up the sky.

Paris is beautiful.

Here's to a good day!

Paris Will Leave Scars   *November 21, 2010*

I think this could forever be my least favorite memory...

As amazing yesterday was, I wish I could say the same about today. Some days are good days and some days are bad. Today was a very, very bad day.

After our delectable breakfast and morning tours of various churches including The Sacre Coeur and other beautiful French landmarks, my brain took a turn for the worse...

We have been riding the subways all week and I have been fine, but today was different. Standing on the side of the tracks, behind the yellow line, waiting for our train to come, I had one of those "out of body experiences". I watched myself walk up to the edge of the tracks, swaying back and forth on the side of the wall, as if trying to stay balanced... and then all of the sudden, I jumped forward. I plummeted into the tracks and within a matter of seconds the train came and it was over.

I snapped out of this daze with my mom pulling me back. I had been mindlessly walking toward the edge as I had been watching myself do.

When it came to me what was happening, I broke down in tears. Unaware of what had just occurred or why, I had a panic attack.
I had to get out of the subway.
Shaking, trembling, crying and scared my mom held me close until the shock passed and I was able to calm down.

The rest of the day I continued to have these "visions" and thoughts but I didn't want to tell anyone and ruin everyone else's vacation. So, I put a smile on my face and told myself that these thoughts were not me and that everything was going to be okay. I created a mantra today... whenever these thoughts come to haunt me I will just tell myself that... *"these thoughts are not me and everything is going to be okay"*

+++++++++

Late afternoon we did something that I have dreamed of doing. We walked up all 2,681 steps of the Eiffel Tower to be greeted by a perfect view of the city.
It was absolutely remarkable!
But I couldn't get the thought out of my head of whether or not I should jump…
This was so dumb though, because you can't jump! There is a cage all the way up the edge, but that didn't seem to matter to my mind. I still thought about jumping…
But, I don't want to, and it's <u>impossible</u>, so why am I thinking about it?
"these thoughts are not me and everything is going to be okay"

++++++++++

After another French aroma filled dinner and dessert, we returned back to the hotel for some good nights rest after a long day. Plus we have to be up early in the morning to be at the train station to catch our train to Amsterdam! We are having Thanksgiving at my grandparent's house in The Netherlands.

++++++++++

I can't sleep tonight.

It's about three a.m. and I am still awake. There are voices telling me that I am going to hurt myself at my grandparent's house. I know this isn't true, but I am scared. Every time I close my eyes I see the noose hanging in my grandparent's shower, but this time, I am hanging from it too… I am sweating, my heart feels like it is going to jump out of my chest and I am terrified.

In tears I woke up my mom. Careful not to wake up my dad or my sister we went to the bathroom, where my mom held me while I cried. I told her everything I had thought all day. I told her that I didn't want to hurt myself but my mind does…why? Am I bipolar? She held me close until I fell asleep, telling me that everything was going to be okay and that I was safe there with her.

I think the Sulfasalazine is making me psycho, but the doctors said that is impossible…

Knowing What To Share
November 22, 2010

My father is now an only child. His only younger brother passed away about two years ago, only days before my birthday.

The last few years have been an extreme hardship on my grandparents and they are so excited to see us for Thanksgiving. Since my Oma had been there with me at the hospital last summer, she often asks how I am doing. My family decided that we should just tell my grandparents that I am feeling fine and that my disease is under control. This is all true; my Ulcerative Colitis is under control.

Why would we burden them with any more stress? I am going to be okay.

My parents and I have decided that I need to stop taking the Sulfasalazine. I can no longer control my thoughts and if this goes on any longer who knows what I could do or what could happen. It's too dangerous.

Already Feeling Better...   *November 24, 2010*

I am feeling so much better! The bad thoughts still come around but I feel like I have some control over them now. I push them out of my mind and tell myself I am stronger than they are.

I need to know for sure what is happening to me. My mom has been trying to call the doctor's office to ask them if they have ever had cases before suffering from similar side effects as me. My doctor is out of the office for vacation and the other doctor on call has never heard of kids having suicidal thoughts when on the medication.

Curious, my mom did an Internet search linking severe mood swings, anxiety, depression and suicidal thoughts to Sulfasalazine; and sure enough, around 1% of people report suicidal thoughts, especially in the first 6 months.

OK, so that is not a high percentage, but it means it is possible. It is possible that the medication is causing me to have these bad thoughts. Those websites only mention the people who reported the problem. Maybe there are even more than that!

Now I am kind of angry. This is a big deal. Why would my doctors not tell me if there were such severe side effects even though the chances are slim… slim or not they are still a possibility and it happened to me!

Thanksgiving With The Dutch November 25, 2010

Today is Thanksgiving!

My grandparents have planned an extravagant party and there are lots of people here, all celebrating this <u>American Holiday</u>, in Europe.

Everyone is so excited! We are calling it "The First Thanksgiving" because for most of the people here, it is.

In Holland, the ovens are very small and are not designed to fit an enormous Thanksgiving beast. My Oma actually faced that dilemma a few weeks ago when she was planning the party; she couldn't find anyone with an oven big enough for our turkey or even a turkey itself. Because Thanksgiving isn't a European holiday, turkeys are not sold in every supermarket in November. The only way Oma could get a turkey big enough for the party was through a good friend who's son was a butcher. Her friend was also able to resolve the other problem because she had a big oven! The turkey barely fit but she cooked it up and brought it to the feast, where we all enjoyed it together.

And... My great uncle is a chef! He made delicious potato dishes, vegetables and custards, pies and deserts of every kind. I must have gained about 10 pounds, but today was a yummy day!

One of the neighbor girls that I have been a friend with for years came to join our party for a while. It was so nice seeing her! As kids, we would ride bikes in the cobblestone streets and play games together. Every time we come back to Holland for a visit, we always make sure to have time set aside to spend with her. I'm so glad I got to see her today!

Home Sweet Home *November 27, 2010*

As fun and exciting this trip was, it was also very emotionally difficult for me. London was breathtaking, Paris was exquisite and Holland was cozy, but I am ready to go to my home now.

It's time to sit back and enjoy our 11-hour flight...

Internet Searches *November 28, 2010*

My mom is frustrated with the doctors. They are not listening to us. So, she is spending lots of time on the computer learning about Ulcerative Colitis. There is a lot of information about ways to heal the colon and cure the disease using diet and supplements. Our doctors never told us any of this…

I am feeling okay…. Except that I have some canker sores in my mouth. This kind of scares me because I had canker sores last summer just before I got sick.

School starts tomorrow and I am so excited to go back to school and see my friends. Ski season is also right around the corner! I am racing again this year and can't wait to start running gates! I just love my new race suit. Bright yellow!

Bloody Nose — *December 2, 2010*

I got a bloody nose yesterday and twice again today. I also have really bad gas! I mean bad, bad farts. I think I am getting sick again... I'm not really eating that much, because I just don't feel like eating. I have no appetite...

School is great! I still haven't told anyone there that I am sick. It is easier when you have a stomachache and throw-up. Everyone understands that, but telling people about bloody diarrhea is a bit awkward.

It Hurts To Move   December 3, 2010

My whole body hurts.

Every limb feels like it weighs 100 pounds and my stomach feels as though a bear went in and scratched up my insides. I hurt.

I am too tired to move or even to attempt getting out of bed. Sitting up once takes about as much effort as 50 sit-ups normally would. Once I get myself to an upright position I am out of breath, dizzy and feel as though I need to lay back down before I fall back down…

I don't think I am going to be able to make it to school today. I can't even gather enough energy to stand up.

This is not a good sign… I might be getting sick again. Since I have been off the Sulfasalazine I have been avoiding certain foods like gluten and dairy that might be aggravating to my colon, but that might not be enough.

Stay Strong

December 4, 2010

My last few entries haven't been so positive. I want to stay positive, but that is hard to do.

I wish I had more happy things to say, but right now I am exhausted. My body is drained and I am just so tired.

But, I haven't even done anything that would make me this exhausted. This is the kind of tired that makes my body hurt all over, when my body feels like it has been through enough and it's just about ready to give up. It takes so much strength and energy to do day-to-day activities that by the time I have completed a regular day, it feels like I spent the whole day running a marathon.

When I woke up this morning, I had to run to the bathroom. And I mean RUN! Something was not right. It started again. The urgency and a little bit of blood in the toilet…

It's hard to think that my disease can come out of remission so easily and that one day I can be happy and healthy and a few days later I can be bleeding when I go to the bathroom.

I am so worn out. My body is so tired of fighting.

Every day is a battle for my body. There is a little war going on inside my body. When I feel sick my mommy tells me to imagine my little warriors and to send them my strength. She says, "Close your eyes and imagine soldiers in your tummy". There is a good side; the side that is going to keep me healthy and fight out all the bad buggies in my tummy, and there is the bad side; the disease. My mom will go on to say "watch while the good guys take over; fight with them; stay strong for them, they can't do this without you". When I hear her say this I remember, this is my battle, I can win this. I have to stay strong for those who matter in my life and for the little soldiers in my tummy who are fighting away the bad guys.

I have to stay strong, because without my resilience, what choice to do I have?

Learning More   *December 5, 2010*

My mom has been reading a lot about Ulcerative Colitis. There is a ton of information about probiotics and different supplements that help the colon. Probiotics are basically the good bacteria in the gut. They help to promote a healthy environment for the gut and help digestion. From what we are reading, when someone has Ulcerative Colitis the good bacteria are decreased and the bad bacteria are increased. So, the goal is to take a whole bunch of the good (pro) bacteria (biotics) to overwhelm the bad bacteria and give the good bacteria a chance to repopulate.

The other thing we have learned from researching my disease is that it is really important to bring down the inflammation in my colon. From what we have been reading, there are some herbs and supplements that might be able to help with that. They include Boswellia Serrata and Aloe Vera. It is kind of cool that frankincense comes from the Boswellia tree because frankincense is one of the gifts that the wise men brought to baby Jesus!

So, since we are afraid of what the Sulfasalazine is doing to my mind, it seems like it is worth it to try some of these ideas that other people write so much about. Our game plan is going to be no dairy, no gluten, no chocolate and lots of probiotics, boswellia and aloe vera.

Let's hope this works!

I Feel Good!

December 9, 2010

I have been taking the probiotics, boswellia, and aloe vera for about three days and I am off all "medication". No more Sulfasalazine or any prescription drugs. We are sticking to my dairy free, gluten free and chocolate free diet along with the supplements and it seems to be helping. I haven't had any pain in the last few days. My trips to the bathroom still occur but they are less frequent and far less blood than before. Things are still not normal but they are better than they were. I'm not expecting a miracle, but there is a chance that this might work.

My scary thoughts still come and go but without taking the Sulfasalazine I feel less nervous that I will do something unintentionally because of the medicine. Bad thoughts still barge into my head and linger in the back of my mind, but without the medicine they are less severe.

Remembering Things....   *December 12, 2010*

When I was in the hospital I remember Dr. Asshole M.D. telling me all about how if this disease didn't get under control it could easily result in having at least part of my colon removed. If the inflammation and the ulcers got too bad, they might need to remove a good portion of my colon, or maybe even all of it as a precaution for colon cancer. He said that he does this surgery all the time and kids do just fine. This is all very scary to think about. If I get my colon removed then I get a colostomy bag, which is a small bag that would hang off the side of my stomach. Because the final track of my digestive system would have been removed it would make it impossible to poop. Therefore my poop would go out a little tube in the side of my stomach and into this bag. I would have to empty the bag, filled with liquid feces, every day and it would be visible to anyone who saw my stomach. Having this would be absolutely awful. I haven't even had my first boyfriend or even kissed a guy, and who would want to kiss a girl with a poop bag hanging off her side. And what about summer, I wouldn't be able to wear my bikini to the lake because everyone would see my colostomy bag...

Thinking about all of this is starting to make me nervous. I don't want to hurt my colon and end up having to remove it. I mean, the Sulfasalazine helped with my disease but it made me crazy, and I can't live that way. Even though I am not on any medicine right now I am not bleeding severely and things seem to be slightly under control. My thoughts just keep spinning about whether or not this is a good idea. The doctor did prescribe the medicine for my disease but he will not listen to me when I tell him it makes me crazy. I had to stop taking it. But I don't want to hurt my colon...

+++++++++

My mom and I talked today about whether or not stopping the Sulfasalazine was a good idea. We talked about how I am nervous and I don't want to hurt my colon by not taking the medicine. To me my health is extremely important, I am going somewhere in my life and I am not going to let some disease hold me back. But, if this disease can either make me crazy or force me to have my body parts removed, well, then I am going to have to learn how to cope with the crazy.

Mind over matter.

It's all in my head anyway, so there must be some way to control it. I know that I don't want to kill myself. I know that the knife on the kitchen counter is not something I would pick up and slice my artery with and I know that the jump rope in the basement will not become a noose. So now, I just need to convince my mind of that.

I will find a way.

Sulfa Is Back

December 14, 2010

So, on the plus side, my farts smell normal! No more vial Shrek farts that could knock out everyone in the room. That is progress. But, the sad news is, I am back on the Sulfasalazine and every bad thought has returned.

I am terrified. The scary suicide thoughts are back and they are uncontrollable. I listen to my music, I meditate, I chant my mantra, I close my eyes and sing a happy song, I don't know what else to do! No matter what I try, the thoughts still linger in the back of my mind.

My happy song is "Do your ears hang low?" It is a kid's song, but when I sing it, I think, *'If their ears are that long they could be used to strangle themselves.'* This is insane! I can't even sing a normal, happy song without thinking up some way to commit such a thing as horrible as suicide. These thoughts won't stop creeping into my mind. When I ride in the car, I stare at the door handle, convincing myself not to open it and roll out.

I told myself I could do this and I am going to. Someway or another I am going to find a way to learn to cope with these thoughts and I am going to live the normal happy life that I want to live.

My mom has started reading this book by a man named, Dr. Dahlman. His book is called "*Why Doesn't My Doctor Know This?: Conquering Irritable Bowel Syndrome, Inflammatory Bowel Disease, Crohn's Disease and Colitis.*" In his book he talks about the need to replace the good bacteria in the gut and the importance of removing all of the foods from one's diet that could be causing an immune reaction against the colon.

Although we decided I should take the Sulfasalazine again we are still researching alternative treatment options. We are not following all of the suggestions in the book, because my GI doctor has told us completely different things. I am still sticking to a restricted diet along with the medicine. We just want to make sure my body is safe while we learn more and decide whether or not these treatment plans will be a safe option for me.

No More Blood!   December 16, 2010

I am still taking the Sulfasalazine. The situation with the crazy mental thoughts has not changed but today, the blood is gone! When I went to the bathroom this morning I saw tiny little rabbit pellets poop, but NO BLOOD. Thank goodness. No blood means the inflammation is going down and my colon is healing. I was so worried about hurting my colon and having it removed, but now that I see a toilet filled with brown instead of maroon and red, I feel much better.

Peanuts and Chocolate are two of my favorite things, but according to my mom's reading, the book says that sticking to the diet restrictions of no dairy and no gluten is not enough. Apparently chocolate and peanuts are a NO, NO, NO, NO, when trying to heal a leaky gut. So, we have to cut those out of my diet too. Bummer!

From reading and researching we have found that "leaky gut" is when someone has "hyper-permeability" in their intestines or bowels. Basically it means that the inflammation of the intestine lining has become more porous which allows food that your body cannot digest to be absorbed into your blood stream. These food particles are recognized as foreign substances and the body forms antibodies against the food and attacks. Your colon gets in the middle of the battle.

The way to help fix this is by cutting out the foods from your diet that the body is fighting against. My mom has found a blood test that helps to identify which foods to avoid so the immune response is decreased and the colon can heal. Since everyone is different, the foods that one can eat another may be sensitive to, hence the reason I have to take the blood test.

"One man's food is another man's poison" (Laucretius)

TAHOE December 20, 2010

This weekend we are staying up in Tahoe with some friends from our race team. Hoping to shred some serious powder. We are here for an awesome ski vacation. We went night skiing last night and when we went to bed the snow started falling! It kept snowing all night. We woke up to eight inches of fresh powder ready to be torn up, but I also woke up to blood and mucus in the toilet.

I am so tired. I want to ski, but my body feels so exhausted and aching that skiing just sounds painful.

We called the doctor, because up until now everything had been fine and I was looking forward to an exciting weekend of skiing with friends, but when I woke to blood and mucus these plans got put on hold. I also have a cold and a very snot-filled nose.

The doctor said to take it easy and I was probably just stressed out and that was why I was bleeding. They say it is normal and that lots of kids with colitis get some colon symptoms when they have a cold. The doctor also said that stressors can cause my disease to flare up and that skiing in cold weather is a big stress on the body, whether I realize it or not. My mom wants me to stay in the hotel room today.

+++++++++

This afternoon, I took a few runs. How could I resist with all the fresh snow? But I was just too tired and my stomach was cramping, so my mommy and I went back to the room.

I tried to be happy at dinner tonight. I don't want our friends to know what is happening with me. We went out for Mexican food but I skipped the flour tortillas, beans, cheese and lettuce. That basically left some dry chicken, a few corn chips and some guacamole. I didn't even want to eat, but I also didn't want to draw attention to the fact that I wasn't eating.

Skiing Makes Me Happy   *December 21, 2010*

Today I skied. Not because I feel that much better, but because skiing makes me happy. If I am supposed to try and decrease my emotional stress, then I need to exercise and just live life. Although they say not to let my disease control my life and not to let it stop me from doing things, sometimes it does. Not that it should but there are those times when because of my disease some things are just not possible that day. But I think that even though I should be "resting and taking it easy" I should also be enjoying life and not be letting my disease control the way I live. So, today I skied.

Crisis Hotline

December 23, 2010

Christmas is supposed to be the happiest time of the year, but for me it's been pretty scary. Things just aren't right.

My mom called the Crisis Hotline today…

My suicide thoughts were really bad last night. I couldn't close my eyes without starting to cry and I got shaking and cold from the absolute fear of killing myself. My mom had to lay with me until I cried myself to sleep. She stayed with me all night and I woke to her holding me this morning. I feel safe when she stays with me. It makes me feel like nothing can happen to me because if I try to do anything she will be there to stop me.

I am scared of being alone.

My dad and my sister do not know about all of this because I don't want to scare them.

From the phone call with the suicide hot line, my mommy got a phone number for a local counselor who could meet with me to try and resolve my suicidal thoughts and ideations. She said she could meet with us right away so today was my first visit.

Before going to the counselor we dropped off my poop samples at the hospital to be tested for any bacteria, parasites or any other abnormalities.

We talked with the counselor for an hour and a half about what I was experiencing and why and how I felt about it. This conversation involved a lot of tissues, because telling someone all about how you want to kill yourself, is not exactly easy for me to say or for my mom to hear. It was a difficult conversation to have with a stranger, but she made me feel better. She said what I am experiencing is something called "intrusive negative thoughts" and she went on to explain the physiology of anxiety disorders. In her description she drew me a picture of a small pathway in the brain that was amplified by my disease and the medicine. Apparently my regular thoughts run on a separate pathway but when something triggers the intrusive thoughts then my mind gets stuck in a loop on that pathway, creating the negative thoughts in my mind. She said the more frequent the negative thoughts, the stronger and deeper the pathway becomes. Because my train of thought gets caught in this loop, it is extremely difficult to get out of, which explains why I have not been able to free my mind of these thoughts.

What she said made sense and going to see her made me feel a whole lot better. It comforted me to know that there is a name for what I am experiencing and that I am not just crazy.

But, my mom and I did something crazy after the appointment...
We went to Taco Bell!

Now, fast food can give anyone diarrhea easily, so tacos when you have leaky gut and Ulcerative Colitis was probably not the best idea, but we didn't think about that until later when it became pretty clear. We get so much conflicting information. One doctor says it doesn't matter what I eat, another says that it totally matters what I eat. One doctor says the medicine cannot cause negative thoughts, another says the negative thoughts are caused by the medicine. One doctor says to try and live as a normal teenager, another says I have to live with all kinds of restrictions. Who do we listen to?

I just wanted to have some fast food and not worry about all my medical restrictions. Everything just seems so futile, like nothing we do even matters at this point.

Christmas With Colitis

December 25, 2010

Christmas is my all-time favorite holiday!

This is my first Christmas with a chronic disease, but that didn't change things, except for the food. No wheat, no gluten, no dairy, no chocolate, no peanuts! We have not done our usual holiday baking this year, because of the restrictions. I kind of miss baking.

Last night on Christmas Eve my mom, sister and I all cuddled up on the couch together and my mom read out loud to us the Christmas classics. My papa sits in his chair and listens to us read the stories aloud. We read "The Grinch", "Wake Up Santa Claus" and "The Night Before Christmas"; all of our favorites! When our stories had been read we hung our stockings above the fire place and made a star for our nativity scene. We hung the star and headed for bed, where thoughts of sugar plums danced in our heads!

This morning, my sister ran into my room at the crack of dawn to inform me that "It's Christmas, Heathy!" and we went to sit at the top of the stairs where we waited for my mom to finish making coffee. When my parents gave us the okay to come down, we were surprised by all the gifts laid out for each of us! The rest of the morning we opened gifts together and shared a wonderful Christmas morning. It is our tradition to have French toast with fruit and orange juice for Christmas breakfast, but because I cannot eat bread we had to improvise. Everyone else still had their Christmas French toast but my mom and I made ours with Gluten Free bread. Although not as good as regular bread, it was good enough for me.

I am just happy it's Christmas and we are all together.

The rest of the day was spent relaxing and enjoying all of the new gifts we had gotten! For dinner we always pick out yummy recipes from our Christmas cookbook, and this Christmas we chose

> *lamb chops*
> *mashed potatoes with glazed hazelnuts,*
> *fire-roasted winter vegetables*
> *baked pears with raspberry sorbet for dessert!*

Instead of using milk in the mashed potatoes we used almond milk.

It was a wonderful day!

It was a very Merry Christmas and the food change was barely noticeable, this diet isn't so bad. I got this!

Merry Christmas to All and to All a Good Night!

My Poop Test Came Back! December 27, 2010

All is good! But in a way, that is bad...
My stool tests came back negative for everything.
Negative for C-Diff
Negative for e-coli
Negative for all parasites

Although it is a good thing that I don't have C-Diff or e-coli or any parasites it would almost be easier if I did. All of those things have a known solution and would be treatable. It would almost be convenient to have come back positive on one of these tests just so we would know for sure what is going on in my body and be able to fix it. But for now, everything still comes back negative.

Blood Labs   *December 28, 2010*

My blood labs were sent out today! They are sending my blood all the way to Florida where they are going to test it for any food sensitivities that I may have. From this we will know for sure what I need to stay away from and what is okay to eat. The exact thing that they are looking for is any IgG antibodies my body has against food. These are not the typical type of food allergy that happens as soon as someone eats something they are allergic to. Symptoms related to food sensitivity with IgG antibodies can occur anywhere from hours up to days after eating something the body reacts to. It is hard to know if food is causing the inflammation in my colon, but it seems worth it to just do the test.

I hope chocolate isn't on the list!

Happy 2011! January 1, 2011

Last night was a fun one! My friend from volleyball stayed the night and we waited up until midnight to celebrate the New Year! We had makeshift fireworks, since they are illegal in our county because of fire hazard. My dad got this firework app on his iPad and we hooked it up to surround sound. He put two iPads on the deck and played fireworks on the loud speakers and displayed them on the screen.

This year is going to be a good one! 2010 was a year of new challenges and new beginnings, but this year, I'm going to figure everything out.

Is It Possible To Be Allergic To All Foods?

January 3, 2011

So, my food sensitivity test came back from Florida and the verdict is….

- Corn
- Egg
- Grapefruit
- Milk
- Mustard
- Orange
- Peanut
- Soybean
- Wheat
- Gluten
- Celery
- Green peas
- Lamb
- Wax Beans
- Hazelnut
- Peppermint
- Swordfish

I don't know if it is possible to be allergic to all foods but if it is, I think I am pretty darn close. This is going to be rough, but I know that it is what I have to do to keep myself healthy. So, starting tomorrow, I eat according to the list.

There is starting to be blood in the toilet again. Not a lot but still, that's not good, so we are hoping that sticking to this diet helps calm things down a little bit until we can figure out what is going on.

I'm not quite sure what I'm going to eat yet, but we will figure something out! We always do...

My mom called the GI doctors again today. They agreed to switch me from Sulfasalazine to Asacol; which is another medicine in the same category as Sulfasalazine. They hope that I will do better on this one. I think they are tired of my mom calling and complaining. Honestly, what else are we supposed to do? I am sick and can't keep living like this. I need to get better, but things just aren't working.

Crisis Counselor   *January 6, 2011*

Today my counselor suggested that we try to identify my stressors (which are the things in life that cause me chronic worry and stress) because she believes that these are contributing to my negative thoughts.

The thing is, my papa and I don't always see eye to eye. We are so alike that we clash sometimes and that leads to arguments and yelling. I don't like arguing with him but he is the person that I argue with most often. I told my counselor about this today and she told me that my dad must be my stressor. She said that arguing with my dad upsets me and when I get upset my brain gets stuck on the negative pathway and then loops around and around and around until it leads to the bad thoughts. She told us that my papa might be my stressor and that he might be to blame for all of these thoughts... This can't be right. I love my papa.

How could this be true? My papa has been in my life since the day I was born and we have always gotten into little squabbles every once in a while, but these scary thoughts just started? *My papa is not the cause.* I do worry a lot. That is true. That's just how I am. I always have been and I probably always will be. But I have never wanted to kill myself because of it... Is this really all connected?

Slalom Race *January 8, 2011*

Today is the first race of the season; Slalom. This is not my best event. We have just finished slipping the course and now everyone is in to refresh themselves before the races start. It is a tight course with a tricky ending, but think I will do okay.

+++++++++

I didn't do as well as I had hoped to. My first run was great but I lost too much time on my second run. I didn't make the podium this race. It was still fun. At the top of the course my coach always has goodies for us right before we reach the start tent. They wax our skis, warm our shoulders, stretch our legs and feed us gummy bears right before our race! It's our team's tradition.

At the race dinner one of the racers also celebrated their birthday and they brought a huge cake; enough for all of the teams to share! Clearly cake has wheat, gluten and eggs, so I didn't eat any but I still got to celebrate with everyone else. Who needs the calories anyway right!? Dinner looked kind of gross so I wasn't too upset that I couldn't eat any. I am starting to get used to always having food with me. We bring a separate meal for me when we go places and just use the microwave. My mom practically brings the whole kitchen when we travel because she worries that I will be hungry – some of the food is good and some is… not so good.

Switcheroo

January 10, 2011

Second semester at school has started. I got a 4.0 for the first semester! But, some things need to change with my class schedule. I am in a home economics class where we make food and learn all kinds of recipes. Crazy thing is that on this diet, I cannot eat a single thing that we make in that class. The last time we made something I didn't eat any and everyone was asking why I wouldn't eat it. I told them I was on a diet and everyone laughed at me and said that I was "too skinny to diet". I tried to explain that it was a medical diet but nobody really seemed to understand. Another complication with this class is that in order to get full credit for the day you have to taste the food that we made in class. But, obviously I can't do that…

So, my mom wrote a letter to the principal explaining my circumstances and saying that I needed to switch out of that class. Our principal was very understanding and he shared with me his personal story. He has experienced serious heart trouble and had to have a heart transplant a few years ago and that is the only reason he is alive today. Sharing this story with me really meant a lot, it made me trust him and feel comfortable going to him if I had any difficulties at school. He told me that he doesn't tell many people that story but he trusts me and felt that I could understand his situation. He told me he had bad days too sometimes and that there are some things that he can't do the same way he used to; he completely understood me wanting to be out of the foods class.

So, he switched me into piano. And this piano class just happened to be the same piano class that the cutest boy in school was in. Lucky me!

Fun Day *January 16, 2011*

I'm still on the Asacol, and now we have added probiotics back into the protocol to help repopulate the good guys in my tummy. I am still on the food restrictions from my IgG blood test but now we have added in NO SUGAR and NO FRUIT for right now because my local doctor thought it would be best to avoid any foods that could promote yeast overgrowth in the gut.

Today was our race team's party at the ice skating rink. All of the families from our team came to skate together: moms, dads, racers, and siblings. We had been skiing and training all day and then we met again at the rink for our party. Everyone was exhausted but we were still ready to have fun and skate; It was a big party! It was hard to walk past the desert table but that is exactly what I had to do. All of those treats and goodies have sugar, eggs, and wheat. Not for me.

I am not liking the newly added restrictions, I am 14 and they are taking sugar away from me?! Oh Boy!

I Hate Breakfast

January 17, 2011

We are learning how to cook and eat new ways, but it is definitely "different". This morning my mom called to me upstairs, "I made cereal for breakfast". I was so excited to hear the word cereal because for the last few days I had been eating strange assortments of vegetables and cardboard toast. I ran down stairs looking forward to my cereal, only to find that is was not cereal. It was amaranth grits. She told me that grits is a kind of cereal… No it's not! Not the kind of cereal I was hoping for. Amaranth grits are gross!

The GI doctors told me that I could eat anything that I wanted and that the food I eat doesn't matter, but that does not seem to be the case. Some days are good days and some days are bad days. Food matters, but I cannot eat this weird food for much longer. It's gross!

Inner Demons?!   *January 20, 2011*

Today was another day with the crisis counselor, but this time things got weird!

She asked me if I had still not told anyone about my condition so I told her about the cutest boy in school and how I had told him a little about how I was feeling both physically and emotionally. Happy that I had found trust in someone she explained that I was making progress.

I am now going to these meetings alone and my mom waits outside. But, today I really wished that my mom were there, because my counselor said something that I had no idea how to answer. She told me again how I have PTSD and how she is quite sure that the pathway in my brain caused by the medicine is what is bringing on all of these negative ideations, but she then said there could also be another cause…
Her exact words were,

> *"It is possible that there are demons in your mind that are trying to talk to you through your thoughts. I would like to speak to these demons next time we meet if that is okay with you."*

Heck no!!!!

This lady is nuts! I don't have demons and she is not about to go all wacko on me and try to talk to my "inner demons"… I can tell you this much, there WILL NOT be a "next time".

Yikes… No more crisis counselor for me!

Trust   *January 22, 2011*

I have come to be very close with the cutest boy in school. He and I have been spending a lot of time together and I trust him. I feel like I can tell him anything and that he will be there for me. He keeps my secrets and he doesn't judge me for my problems. That's why, I told him...

I told him about my disease and my time in the hospital and what was wrong with me. I told him about how I have sad thoughts sometimes and how I am extremely sensitive, but it's because I am scared. I am scared of things changing, of him leaving and hurting me.

But I trust him.

I need to have someone who is there for me besides my family. Although I can always turn to my family when something is wrong. I need someone else, a friend that I can rely on, and that friend is this boy. I know he will be there when I need him... I trust him.

Winter Concert   *January 25, 2011*

Tonight was a very special night for me.

My sister had her winter concert for violin at my school tonight. The cutest boy in school was also at the concert, so we were both there…

At intermission I went to find him, but he found me first!
It was raining pretty hard outside, but we didn't care, we went out there anyway and sat on the edge of the building and talked. After a few minutes of talking he leaned in to kiss me!

My heart was racing! I didn't know what to do. I had never kissed a boy before and he was just so cute! My butterflies were going crazy, but I leaned in to kiss him back! I thought we were going to have a little peck of a kiss, but no…. there was tongue! Tongue? What do I do with tongue!? I had no idea what was happening, or what to do…so I just let him kiss me. Apparently I have a lot to learn… but it was still romantic. My first kiss, at a winter concert, in the rain, with the cutest boy in school… perfect!

He doesn't care that I am a little complicated… he kissed me!

Asacol Not Working...   *January 26, 2011*

I think I am getting worse. I have been on the Asacol and have also stuck to my dietary restrictions, but things do not seem to be improving. There is still blood in the toilet and the frequency in having to run to the bathroom has gone up to about 12 times a day.

I honestly just don't understand. I feel frustrated and confused. I have done everything that the doctors told me, and they promised that this medication should work and that my disease should be under control shortly, but it's not. I have stuck to the diet <u>and</u> I have been taking my medicine, yet still, bloody diarrhea. How can I be doing what they say will make me better, but be getting worse?

Where Is My Hair Going? January 31, 2011

I've been home all day today. School was really just not an option today. I have serious sinus congestion, I feel like I am drowning in my own snot, I have horrible back pain and to make matters worse, I also have extremely bloody diarrhea and a constant sharp pain in my stomach.

I can't just be like other teenagers and have a cold. Because my immune system is so whacked, when I get a small cold or something like that I also get an increase in all my disease symptoms. So every time I get sick, I get hit hard, and double hard, with the sickness and the disease. This is to be expected the doctors say…

I spent a lot of time showering and steaming out my congestion today but I noticed that every time I showered I left a large hairball in the drain. My hair is falling out. When it dries, it doesn't dry normally. It dries brittle and sharp, like hay. Then if I touch it my hair will break and fall out. My ponytail has lost about half its thickness of hair.

My hair is falling out!

Race Day   February 5, 2011

I had diarrhea this morning, but I am determined to race.

Today is our home race. We are hosting a Giant Slalom race; which is my all time favorite! My family, along with all the other race families, need to be at the ski area by 7AM to register and get our race numbers. I have been training for this race for weeks, and I am ready to tear it up! All last night I was laying in bed racing the course in my head, studying the course and preparing myself for the race.

There is one girl who is the girl to beat. She is on my team and she is really good, but I am pretty good too… She just always beats me in practice. But today, I am determined to win!

Victory is mine!

++++++++++

I beat that girl and took the race with first place! I also had another surprise waiting for me at the podium. At our home race, every year, our team gives out an award called the "little e award" in memory of one of our young racers who passed away not too long ago. The award symbolizes leadership, dedication and support for the team and for the sport. I was given this award tonight. My coaches wanted to honor me for my hard work as a racer and for always being there to support my teammates and make every occasion just that much more fun. It was an honor. Little e's parents even came to personally congratulate me. Wow!

++++++++++

That award made up for dinner. The team arranged for a local Chinese restaurant to provide dinner to all of the racers. We should have talked to the cook at the restaurant before tonight! Everything was cooked in soy sauce. I had white rice and some left-over chicken my mom had brought from home.

Holistic Medicine Here We Come February 8, 2011

Holistic doctors are supposed to be able to treat a patient using herbs and natural remedies instead of drugs from the pharmaceutical companies. Apparently there are a lot of the same chemicals in plants that act as medication. Therefore these holistic doctors treat diseases using natural remedies.

At this point I am ready to try anything. This whole holistic thing sounds kind of crazy to me, but lots of people, websites and magazines say that it has proven to work on millions of people, so I guess it's worth a shot.

Our appointment isn't for a few hours but I am not looking forward to going. I am beginning to lose faith in doctors. I am Angry. I have done everything that I am told to do and I am not getting better. If this disease is as common as they say it is then why am I still sick and bleeding and nobody can figure out how to stop it? I want to hear the truth from my doctors. If I am that one in a million case, then I want to know. If they can't help me, I want to know, instead of putting my faith and my health in their hands when they are unsure about what to do with it.

+++++++++

I'm not really sure what to think about how the appointment went. We talked about my bloody poop and my tummy aches the way we do at every appointment:

"describe your stool to me", "does this hurt?", "how are you today?"

"Yes it hurts. I am bleeding out my butthole, my intestines are torn to pieces; so when you push on them it doesn't feel too great, I feel like I am carrying satin's child inside my body and nobody can figure out what's wrong. So… I'm doing just dandy today, that's why I am here. How are you?"

His holistic approach was barely different then what I have heard before. He told me to stop drinking tea and eating potatoes. Wonderful, now that I barely have any food left in my diet, why not take out tea and potatoes too. Maybe if I just live on water and rice for the rest of my life, I won't have bloody diarrhea anymore. Sounds wonderful. Like every other doctor he ordered blood labs and stool samples. Once again, the lab tests are looking for parasites and bacteria…I hope they find some.

No More Asacol *February 10, 2011*

Physically, I feel worse. I have been on the Asacol for six weeks now and there has been no improvement whatsoever, if anything I have gotten dramatically worse. Bloody, explosive diarrhea; literally explosive and so bloody that the bowl looks black. I also poop out the pills; whole. If I look in to the dark blood-stained toilet bowl, amongst the slight food remnants, there are small red pills. I am pooping out my pills. So, I swallow them and then just poop them out; does that mean they aren't even doing anything at all?

I stopped taking the Asacol. If anything I have gotten so much worse on this medicine that it would almost be better to just not take anything than to take it right now. But, doing nothing would be dangerous. The holistic doctor suggested that instead of the Asacol we return to taking the boswellia and probiotics. We also added in digestive enzymes and glutamine. Both of which are supposed to help with breaking down food and improving digestion. I am still following my STRICT dietary restrictions from the IgG list and not eating potatoes or tea, as suggested by the holistic doctor. This is all just craziness. How can one little disease be so hard to figure out?

Normal?

February 13, 2011

I have been off the Asacol for all of three days, and guess what… normal poop! How is this possible? A medicine that was supposed to make me better actually made me worse, twice?!

As of right now seeing a normal poop in the toilet is something that deserves a celebration and a jump for joy. I called my mom to come and look! The true excitement that can come from pooping out a normal log is unimaginable when you have Ulcerative Colitis.

I almost forgot what it felt like to poop!

Since what we are doing right now, with the probiotics, bosewellia and digestive enzymes seems to be working, why would we stop doing it! So, we plan to continue and to also maintain the diet in hopes that the combination will keep the normal poops coming my way!

I've Got The Munchies!   *February 16, 2011*

I am so hungry!!
How long will I have to eat this way?
I hope it's not forever.

I just want life to go back to the way it was before I was sick. When I could live like a normal kid and eat like one too! I want to be able to go out with my friends and not have to worry about food. My friends all go out to parties every once in a while and half of them don't even drink. But, I am scared to go to a party. The idea of drinking or smoking or anything like that terrifies me. I need control of my body. The thought of not having control of my actions or my thoughts scares me, because I don't know what will happen; and not knowing makes me nervous. These last few months I have had barely any control over what happens to my body or my health.

I feel like I am maturing faster than some of the other kids I go to school with. Maybe it is because I have faced these challenges at such a young age, or maybe it is just because I am realizing the true sacredness of life and how it deserves to be lived out to its fullest, because you never know when it could be taken away.

My life changed over night. I never really thought that was possible and I certainly never thought that it would happen to me. But it did, and I have to move on from it and learn how to create a new life in a way that I can live, because I can't live my old life anymore. Things will never be the way that they were before I got sick, but who is to say they won't be better. Maybe this disease will bring out parts of life I never even knew existed.

Early Morning Fiasco *February 21, 2011*

It's an early morning training day for the race team, which means they open the lifts just for the team at 7AM before anyone else is even there. The coaches set up a SuperG course and we run it until the lifts open. Then it is taken down and we share the mountain with everyone else.

Not only did my morning start out with a tight race suit and frozen chair lifts but it also started with a scary thing that happened, a tantrum, and hysterical crying. I was riding the frozen chair with one of the youngest players on our team. She was sandwiched between my friend and me when all of a sudden she slipped off the chair lift. We grabbed her coat and pulled as hard as we could to bring her butt back onto the chair. I don't even know how we did it! I don't even know how we didn't all fall off the chair! There was no time to think. We just had to react.

After that we raced really well. High on adrenalin, I think. Then I had a panic attack.

There was a pancake breakfast for all the racers after our early morning training but I couldn't eat any. Just because I couldn't eat the pancakes didn't mean that I couldn't smell them cooking, watch the syrup be slowly poured over them, or see everyone else around me eat them. It all just got too overwhelming. All of the smells around me that I couldn't enjoy but was expected to sit next to and pretend didn't exist. I couldn't handle it. I broke down in tears. I was sad. All I wanted was a pancake.

After breakfast I went back out to train but didn't last long. After only a few more runs down the course I came back inside and sat in the lodge with my mommy. I just don't feel good today. I am discouraged and sad and along with that my tummy hurts. Today, I think I just need to lay low.

When we got home this afternoon my mom spent hours in the kitchen cooking up some kind of meal. I wasn't sure yet what she was making until she called me down to eat.

Pancakes, she made pancakes!

These were not regular pancakes. They were made with oats and amaranth and were honestly pretty disgusting, but I didn't care. The fact that she put so much effort in to make me pancakes after she saw how upset I was at breakfast, warmed my heart. This reminded me that I am not in this alone. My family is right here by my side and we are going to fight this together, no matter how long it takes, we are going to win this battle. WE can do this!

++++++++++

Tennis season starts on Monday and I can't be more excited! Hoping to play on varsity I can't wait to start hitting again. I am not going to let my disease get in the way of tennis season. I am aware that there are going to be days that I don't feel good or just can't make it to practice, but I will be there, working hard every day that I can! I promise myself that.

Papaya Seeds   *February 22, 2011*

I am still not on any medicines; just the supplements – and the diet. Never forget the diet.

Some days are good poop days and some days are not so good poop days. But there are no days as bad as when I was on the Asacol. No more explosive diarrhea or blood so black it looks like tar. Now, a bad day is a little bit of blood on the tissue or a little bit in the toilet water. The blood is red now, but in comparison to what was happening before, this is still improvement.

We went back to the holistic doctor today and he told us something crazy. He prescribed a short burst of steroids to get the inflammation down to stop the little bit of bleeding. This made sense and I am willing to do the short burst of Prednisone, but what he said next was the crazy part. He told me that papaya seeds were a natural anti-parasitic and that if I had any parasites in my gut the papaya seeds would help to kill them. Yet, he doesn't want me to just swallow some papaya seeds as if they were pills, No, he wants me to chew five seeds a day... I wonder how that's going to taste?

There was some good news from this appointment though. He told me that there was a certain type of bread that was free of gluten and wheat but tastes good. It is called Spelt Sourdough. Yippee!! Toast!!

+++++++++

After the appointment we went straight to the store and bought this Spelt Sourdough, went home and toasted it up. He was right; it tasted like normal bread, just a little more dense! I am in heaven!

We also bought papayas and tested out the seed chewing right away. Well, chewing up papaya seeds is gross! They are bitter and hard and made my tongue feel numb, but this is all part of it. As crazy as it sounds, it could work. I mean who am I, to judge what could work and what couldn't. The medications that we hoped would work had failed, so might as well try some crazy ideas. What's the worst that could happen?

SuperG Weekend   March 5, 2011

Today is a SuperG race at a resort about 4 hours away from home. Last night my dad and I drove up here to the resort, just the two of us. My mom and my sister aren't coming to this race because Merel is sick. We packed up a bunch of 'Heather Food' and brought stuff so that my dad can cook meals while we are here. But I think this will be a good weekend because as of right now I am pooping normal and I think if I can stick to my diet all weekend that should remain the case.

On our way here last night we met up with some other race families at a bar and grill for dinner. Prepared, my dad took out the hamburger that my mom had made for me. This burger consisted of buffalo meat, lettuce and two slices of spelt toast as a bun. To make my burger taste better, I salted each bite before eating it. Thinking that nobody was paying much attention to me eating I just ate my burger and listened peacefully to the conversation. Then, one of the other racer's dads leaned over and said, "You want some burger with that salt?"

Ha-ha! Very funny, jerk.
I know he doesn't understand but as if I didn't stick out enough with my weird burger, I didn't need him to point out my eating habits. I am well aware. Hearing him say that hurt my feelings, because I know that I eat weird, but I hoped that people didn't notice or didn't care. When he brought it up at dinner, it made it clear that he noticed and decided to make a joke. I didn't think it was funny.

All In Moderation
March 10, 2011

Today my mommy called the doctor in Florida who did my food sensitivity testing, because I still flare up occasionally and we are unsure why. He told us that we have to be sure to rotate my food and no single food should be repeated two days in a row. If I do start eating foods too frequently my body could form a reaction against food that I eat a lot and then we would have to cut that food out of the diet. At least for a while until my body is ready to have it reintroduced.

Given the circumstances, and the extremely limited amount of foods that I can eat, it is going to be extremely difficult to find enough foods to fill up a week, without repeating foods. The doctor suggested that we make a food schedule with a list of what food I can eat on what day, to make things easier. Easier? This isn't going to be easy… we are going crazy! As if it isn't hard enough to have so few food options, now I can't eat them too close together and I have to schedule out what food is okay for what day? This is nuts! My mom got really sad today. I think she is feeling overwhelmed by all of this.

To get a second opinion before we started this rotation thing (which is going to make our busy lives really difficult) my mom called up the Holistic doctor and asked his opinion on the idea. He too agreed with the rotation idea, which finalized the plan. On top of agreeing to the rotation he also told my mom that my stool tests came back with high levels of bad bacteria. He ordered a short course of Ciprofloxacin (an antibiotic) to help kill these bacteria in order to create a healthier environment for the good bacteria in my gut.

So, we came up with a food rotation schedule. It's going to be rough, and I'm sure I am going to begin to hate all of this food after a while. But hey, it's worth a shot, right?

All Hell Breaks Loose   March 18, 2011

Maybe the Ciprofloxacin was a bad idea. I think instead of just killing the bad bacteria, it might have taken out the good guys too. Basically, all hell broke loose. Bloody, explosive, urgent diarrhea, too many times a day to even count…

Panicked, my mommy called the GI doctors today.

They said that I need to be back on the Asacol and sent an order into the pharmacy.
This is so infuriating and frustrating. WHY WON'T THEY LISTEN TO US?!

The Asacol made me sick, really sick, way worse than I ever was before; and they want to put me back on it?! I felt terrible when I was on the Asacol. Everything hurt, my hair was falling out, I was loosing a significant amount of blood daily, I was losing weight and my disease was getting worse. Who in their right mind would put someone back on a medication that was causing all of these things to happen? I can't believe this, what kind of doctors are these people?

What Is Happening?   March 23, 2011

Today was a terrifying day.

I got a call at school saying that I needed to be dismissed. I didn't know why or where I was going until my mom called me. She told me not to worry and that everything was going to be okay, but we needed to go to the hospital right away. The hospital is about three hours away and she told me we would be staying down there for a few days.

I didn't know what was happening. I was scared.

The class that I was pulled out of to receive this phone call happened to be piano, the class I had with the cutest boy in school. I was crying when I talked to my mom and I was nervous. When I returned to class, he could tell that something was wrong; he sat with me on the piano bench and talked to me. I explained to him that I would be going to the hospital for a few days and I didn't know much else, but I assured him he didn't need to worry, because I was going to be okay… I hope.

There is another boy though… He has bright red hair and he's very sweet. This boy has a pretty big crush on me, but unfortunately I don't feel the same way. He too saw my teary eyes and also asked what was wrong. I told him less, but I explained that I had to go to the hospital; did not say why or that I was sick though.
He seemed worried, so I told him it was no big deal and that everything would be fine. This wasn't true, maybe it was a big deal, and maybe everything wasn't going to be fine… but I didn't know for sure and I really didn't want to make a scene at school.

The cutest boy in school came up and gave me a big, tight hug. He told me everything was going to be okay and that he would see me when I got back.

On the drive down my mom talked to me about how the doctors think my situation is getting too dangerous and that we need to stop the bleeding right away. For the last few days I have been bleeding quite a bit and have also had a lot of mucus in my poop. I am taking the medicine, but it is not helping. There is a storm expected to hit our town this weekend and they wanted me to come down right away, before the storm, so that is why we had to leave from school. I am very sick right now - I know that.

It is time to see the GI doctors. That was why we had to rush to them today... But we won't actually see them until tomorrow.

My family still has our old house so that is where my mommy and I are staying tonight. But, I'm nervous about tomorrow. I don't want them to admit me again...

The Appointment

March 24, 2011

The doctors don't listen. They don't seem to even care that the Asacol makes me deathly ill; they just tell me to keep taking it and to add to it they also prescribed me steroids. So now I am on Prednisone and Asacol and we are sticking with taking the Probiotics as well.

The specialists told my mommy that sometimes families opt for surgery because it is easier than all of the medications and "flares". They said that sometimes only a small part of the colon may need to be removed and the cut ends can be stitched together. That way someone can still poop. If more needs to be taken, then they make this pouch inside and there is just watery diarrhea. If those don't work or the intestine wall is too damaged then the only true solution would be to remove the entire colon and receive a colostomy bag.

NO WAY.

Why won't they listen? How am I supposed to trust these doctors and get healthy again if they will not listen to me when I say that the medicine makes me sick.

Roller-coaster Ride

April 29, 2011

I've been too tired to write in my journal for the past month.

It's been a roller-coaster ride. I am better one day and sick the next. Still sticking to the diet and I am following the doctors instructions exactly, but SURPRISE just like we told them, the medicine makes me sick.

I don't know if it is me, or the medicine, or the disease, but things are not working the way that they are supposed to be working. I am frustrated, sick and upset.

It is not as bad as it was before but I am still bleeding, and I should not be bleeding anymore. This is not okay. I also have really bad sinus congestion, the way I did the first time I had gone on the Asacol. But what does it matter? The doctors won't listen.

Today my mom called the GI specialists again to let them know that I was still sick. They asked how many days of school I had missed. What? I don't miss school. I want to go to school. When I am with my friends, I feel happy. If I am home alone, all I can think about is how bad I feel. Besides, I like school. I get good grades and only a few people even know that anything is wrong.

After much debate they decided to switch me off of the Asacol and onto something called Balsalazide, which is another anti-inflammatory drug. Finally they are listening to us; that took way too long! They hoped this one would be better - third time is a charm. I can't believe they just now decided to listen to what we had to say, after months of me and my mom complaining they just now decide that maybe the medicine isn't working. Wow! The doctors said that with the Balsalazide it would take about 2-3 weeks for the medicine to take any affect and that it would take at lest 4 weeks for my poop to be normal again.

I guess that's better than getting worse. The wait is better than never!

Volunteering At The Fair Grounds   *April 30, 2011*

I spent the afternoon running around in very uncomfortable shoes, a black skirt and itchy white button down; I was a caterer for a school benefit dinner.

The event was actually pretty fun. Serving food, selling raffle tickets and getting to talk to everyone at the table that I was serving and getting to meet new people in the community. Plus we made a bunch of money for our school; it was a great success!

Having to know were the bathroom was at all times, and making a run for it only twice was the flip side of the night. With Ulcerative Colitis, my number one concern anywhere I go is, "where is the closest bathroom and how fast can I make it there?"

Only once was my escape to the bathroom slightly awkward. I was serving a table and I got "the feeling". I thought, "oh no, this is horrible timing" but there really is nothing I can do besides run for it. So, I ended the conversation in saying, "I forgot something I will be right back" and then literally, started running towards the small bathroom in the back of the fair grounds hall. Thankfully nobody was in there to hear me explode into the toilet and I made it. It was close, and even though it was probably pretty embarrassing to have to leave the table and then have everyone see me frantically running for the bathroom door, I did what I had to do and it was a far better outcome then letting her rip in my catering skirt...

Tennis　　　　　　　　　　　　　　　　　　May 4, 2011

Right now, things seem to be improving but, ever so slightly. I am not as congested anymore but the cramping is getting worse. When I play tennis my stomach will tighten up and make me feel like I need to go to the bathroom. Now I have a slight ability to "hold it" that I didn't have before, which is also improvement believe it or not. So when I play tennis and get this feeling, I just try to hold it, which results in more cramping and pain. Sometimes I just say I need water and go sit down for a minute until the pain passes.

Why don't I just go to the bathroom when I get this feeling? Well… the bathrooms up by the tennis courts are locked, and nobody can seem to find the key. The closest bathroom is in the gym, which is down a hill, through the parking lot and past the baseball field… I wouldn't make it.

I am just trying to stay positive. I am thankful for my newfound talent of being able to hold my urge to poop, making running to the bathroom less awkward. Now I can clench my cheeks and make a nice slow walk to the stall. Tennis is also going great; I am playing varsity mixed doubles as a freshman and still have a 4.0 in school! At least most parts of my life are going smoothly even though the health parts are still a little bumpy.

Don't dwell on the bad; be thankful for the good!

It's Bumpy Again   May 12, 2011

This journal is a place for me to vent, and talk about what is happening in my life. I don't really write in my journal when things are going good, it is more of a place for me to lay off the burden when things are not going so well, like today.

I stayed home from school today. It was another morning where it hurt to get out of my bed. Every muscle was sore and it took so much energy to sit up that by the time I had, I needed to lie back down again. My run to the toilet reached six this morning, <u>before</u> I was about to leave for school. That is six times of bloody, explosive, urgent diarrhea in one hour. That is about five too many, and we decided that maybe school wasn't such a good idea. I spent the next hour or so crying my eyes out. I am tired and stressed and just can't handle this anymore. "Why me?" I ask myself. As a child I ate healthy, exercised and was as happy as could be. I am nice to people, friendly and outgoing. Why does this have to happen to me?

I am just tired, and need to cry. I can't really explain why I am sad; maybe because I poop blood so many times a day or my stomach hurts all the time and I can't eat anything, but that really isn't it. I am not crying because I am in pain or hungry. I am crying because I am tired, stressed and scared. Tired of being sick, scared of getting worse and stressed that life isn't as carefree as it used to be.

I am still on the Balsalazide and am taking VSL#3 probiotics along with digestive enzymes. My dietary restrictions are still in order and I am following them as closely as possible, although I have started eating wheat once in a while. Imagine being a teenage girl and not being able to eat anything yummy. It really is horrible! I want to be normal and have fun and eat yummy things the way other kids my age do, but that isn't an option right now. Bread is as close to normal as I can get, and it's only once a week. But that one bread-day every week is like a day sent from heaven! I look forward to my slice of spelt sourdough and butter!

Still Not Helping?   May 15, 2011

I know the doctors told me that it would take a while for this medicine to start working but I feel like things really haven't changed much. I'm just not feeling any better. My bathroom run has made it down to about eight times a day. Things are much worse in the morning and at night, which is good. My bowels are less active during the day when I am at school, making things easier, so then I don't have as many uncomfortable situations at school.

It is actually kind of interesting… Every single morning, without fail, as soon as I open my eyes (that moment when your eyes open and your body realizes that it's morning) my stomach gets the memo that it is now morning. Then, I get "the feeling" and have to Run, Run, Run, to the bathroom. EVERY MORNING. My sister knows now that when my bedroom door opens the toilet better be free and there better not be any obstacles in the way, because I am on my way there!

New Doctor!
May 19, 2011

New doctor – different hospital. Hoorah!

He is a very kind man, I actually feel like maybe he really does care about me and my health. With the other doctors I have felt like I am just another patient with another problem that they have to fix. The specialists that I originally had, well, I actually felt like I was annoying them. Like since I was a complicated case, and nothing seemed to work for me that I was annoying to them because I just had to make things complicated. I didn't mean to be that one in a million person that nothing worked for… I just am.

This doctor makes me feel like that is okay and like I don't need to be sacred anymore because he can help me. I really hope that's true!

The new doctor; he actually listened to us! He heard what we had to say and he didn't care about my past or all the things I had been told before. All he cared about was now. He wants to move forward toward a healthy future. We were starting over with a clean slate and a new doctor.

The appointment today went really great.

He suggested that we resume with the Asacol and this time add more prednisone. Explaining that sometimes we need to bring down the inflammation with prednisone before the Asacol can work. Although we have had problems with Asacol in the past and swore to never use it again, he made sense. And I trust him. He honestly seems like a good man who really wants to help. So, we agreed to the prednisone and the Asacol, once again.

This new doctor also told us that while on prednisone what I eat really doesn't matter. He said not to worry about any further dietary restrictions and to practice "moderation only".

No Progress — May 24, 2011

The diarrhea and bleeding are not improving at all. I am still worse in the morning and in the evening. Why aren't things changing? I am on steroids and medicine…

My mommy called the nice doctor today and told him that things just aren't looking good. Nothing has changed, and by now things should have already started improving. The doctor understood and told us to stop taking the Asacol but to continue with the Prednisone until we figured something out.

Progress, Finally!   May 27, 2011

My frequency has gone WAY down and things are actually looking up. I even had one tiny little poop today and I mean tiny, like a single little baby carrot in the toilet. But hey, that is progress. I was so excited to see this little poop! My mom came upstairs to see it and we celebrated my poopy! Thank goodness! This is the first poop I have had in a long time. Every little poop counts.

I am heading off to the Sober Grad party at my school. Basically, this is a big party that the school puts on after graduation with bounce houses, velcro walls, poker, dancing, a beauty salon and all kind of fun stuff! It goes until 4AM and it's just one big fun party to celebrate graduation. I am excited! My friends and I are all going together after the ceremony! Can't wait!

The bounce house probably isn't something that will go in my favor so I think I will steer clear of it. My intestines don't really like to be shaken up, and when they are, they let me know they don't like it with an urgent trip to the potty.

Overall, today is a good day: good poop and a party!

Prednisone Sucks   May 30, 2011

When someone is on Prednisone at a high dose for a while, things start to really be a bummer.

It makes my cheeks puff up like a chipmunk, I get a little fat deposit at the bottom of my tummy and basically just get "puffy" everywhere. Also, I get cranky and have hot flashes, cold flashes, flushed face, dry skin, water retention, increased nerves, increased hunger, increased risk of infection, trouble sleeping, and muscle/ joint pain. Now, these are only the side effects that I have come to be familiar with. Whenever a doctor says "we are going to start you on a short burst of prednisone" I immediately think, "Yippee, just what I wanted, to be fat, itchy, cranky and hot all right before summer starts; perfect". Prednisone is honestly one of my least favorite things in the entire world. It just makes me feel like (for lack of a better word) crap.

Now, lucky for me these are the only symptoms that I really experience, but having a fat tummy, chipmunk cheeks and a bright red face are not things that go unnoticed. Neither is being cranky or wanting to eat everything in sight. But it could be worse, since some of the other side effects of Prednisone include, Excess Stomach Acid Secretion, Bleeding of the Stomach or Intestines (which would be a really inconvenient side effect for someone with Ulcerative Colitis), Small Red Skin Lesions caused by Dilated Blood Vessels, Diabetes, Osteoporosis, High Blood Sugar, etc.

Overall, Prednisone sucks.

Colonoscopy Day   June 2, 2011

This morning, my mom, papa and I woke up at the crack of dawn to get to the hospital (which is more than 2 hours away) for my Colonoscopy. The doctors want to look around my colon to see what exactly we are dealing with right now and the only way to find out exactly what is going on in there, is to go in there.

++++++++++

Lying down on the table in my backless gown, I waited for the anesthesiologist to come in to meet me. I wanted to meet my anesthesiologist because if you think about it, the biggest risk of a colonoscopy lies in the hands of the anesthesiologist. They are really the only one in this process who could kill me; therefore I want to meet them and make sure they are someone I trust with my life.

My anesthesiologist came in happy to meet me and reassured me that everything would go smoothly. He seemed like a good guy. A few minutes later the nurse came in and started my IV. Then shortly after that the anesthesiologist came back in and put the anesthesia straight into my IV. I watched as the room went fuzzy then they pushed me though the double doors in to the surgery room where I laid on the table and watched as the doctor grabbed the big long tube he was about to stick down my throat so that I could breathe. But I was still awake! I couldn't get up the energy to say that I was awake but I was! My heart started to race; I don't want any tube going down my throat while I'm awake! That's the last thing I remember, so, I guess I fell asleep in the nick of time!

When I woke up in the recovery room my mommy and papa were right by my side. My mom says I looked over at her and said, "mommy you look like pooh bear." She had on a nice white shirt and black slacks, but the shirt was a little too short.

My fingers fascinated me because I swear; I saw rainbows coming out of each finger. One of the nurses walked past my room and I called for her to come in, "look at my fingers" I told her "there are rainbows coming out of them". She laughed and so did I, uncontrollably. I then said "Hi" to every other nurse that walked passed my room and waved my rainbow hands at them. My popsicle intake reached about 12 because they told me that I could have as many popsicles as I wanted in the recovery room, so I took advantage of that and had one of each flavor. Then when I decided root beer was my favorite, I just kept eating them. I talked and laughed and told stories to each and every person in earshot. The nurses were all laughing and told my parents that I had been one of the funniest kids they had ever seen come off of anesthesia. I guess I made their day.

Apparently the actual test didn't go so well and the inflammation extends from my rectum all the way to the furthest portion of my colon. My doctor said he did not expect to see this much inflammation when on both Asacol and Prednisone. He talked to my parents for a long time and suggested to stay off the Asacol long term while continuing with Prednisone and probiotics – at least for now. The next stage of medications needs to be considered.

The Farm   June 20, 2011

It has been just over a year since I first got sick. My mom and papa decided to take a few days to go to a super fancy saxophone store in Las Vegas. My papa is so excited to get a new saxophone! My sissy and I are staying at our friend's house for a few days. These friends live on a farm.

Yesterday was our first day here and they took us into town for lunch. We spent the rest of the day just helping out at the farm and relaxing. The kids are fun and the family is so sweet, but my sister and I are just not exactly accustomed to farm-life.

After the chores, we went swimming at a small lake near their house. I know that they all noticed that I have put on weight since ski season. I thought, *"If anyone asks me, I will probably blow my top. I know that I am fat! That's what the Prednisone does, but really, you have to ask about it?"* Fortunately, I had my answer ready, just in case. I was prepared to answer with a smile and say, *"I'm on a medicine that makes me fat - end of story."* Thank goodness I never had to say it!

After our day at the lake - me spending it being self-conscious about my pudge - we went back to the house for a delicious meal that we all enjoyed. After a long day, I went straight to sleep.

Puking All Day — June 21, 2011

Today we got to come home. My dad came to get us at about noon from the farm. Yet, the moment he pulled in the drive, my sister exploded bright pink vomit all over their garage. Then, moments later one of the other kids threw up. Gross. When we were driving home, it was my turn and I said "pull over!" My dad pulled over immediately as I stuck my head out of the car and puked all over the side of the road, then my sister did the same – again.

Needless to say, we are spending the rest of the day in bed. The family we stayed with called and said that all of them are also throwing up. FOOD POISONING. Fantastic. As if my gut hasn't been through enough this past year.

Colorado   *July 2, 2011*

It's been an adventure already. After having our car over heat on the pass and having the cutest cowboy ever pull over to help us, we had to leave our car at a random auto shop in Reno and race to make our train; which ended up being 12 hours delayed. We decided to kill 12 hours in Reno by eating appetizers, entrees and desserts at different restaurants. We walked then ate. Then walked again to a different restaurant and ate the next course. For dessert, I had the most amazing, decedent chocolate cake. One good thing about Prednisone is that I am eating whatever I want. We finally made our 24-hour train ride, and now, we are in Colorado for our family reunion.

Today we went on an awesome hike. A big group started this hike, and half way into it all but four of those people bailed. My papa, uncle, cousin and I were the only ones who made it to the top!

On the way down, there was this horse. My cousin who had made it to the top with me started being chased by this wild horse. We ran, yelling mean words at the terrifying horse, hoping not to be trampled. As soon as we jumped the fence we knew we were fine and sat on our truck waiting for my papa and uncle. About 20 minutes later, as we were baking in the sun, my mom and my aunt come prancing down the trail, with the horse from hell. We wondered, "What are they doing with that horse?"

They had found the horse and an abandoned saddle. As they approached, this trailer pulled up and two cowboys go out. They saw the horse and said, "Hey mam, is that your horse?" My aunt answered, "No, we just found it." The cowboy went on to say, "Oh, well I have been missing my horse and I believe that is her." But we could tell that the horse did not like him because the horse wouldn't approach him! Hmm… suspicious… The cowboys started being rude because we were hesitant to give them the horse. We are pretty sure that it wasn't their horse. Maybe they were horse thieves! After handing over the horse, we took the number from their license plate, just in case.

As if the hike and the horse weren't enough we decided to head off on another adventure. All the kids went to play hide and seek in the woods; with the dogs. This was all fun and games until we heard the dog yelp in pain. A deer jumped out of the bushes and started charging at all of us. We ran for our lives up a steep hill and all 15 of us made it over the fence just as the deer was approaching. Looking back at how steep the hill was and how high the fence was, I don't know how we did it, must have been adrenaline! Anyway, the dog was bleeding because the deer kicked him! Thankfully he kicked the dog and not any of us.

My aunt is taking the dog to the vet now and as for the rest of us, I think we will call it a day.

The 4th of July

July 4, 2011

I'm tired today. My whole family is heading into the town of Steamboat to celebrate the holiday and watch the fireworks, which should be fun. I've been eating whatever I want this trip, which is nice for a change but I just feel low. Maybe because the last few days have been a nonstop adventure. With my family I should be used to that.

We went to town and my mom got in a bit of a tangle with my aunt, because I wasn't feeling good and my aunt just kept saying, "Oh she's fine, just get some food in her." But really, I wasn't fine. When I get low and tired, that usually means that something is wrong inside, but since I am on the prednisone we have no way of knowing. My mom got annoyed that my aunt kept saying that and she gave her a piece of her mind. Nobody understands why I get so tired.

When it came time for the fireworks I really wasn't looking forward to loud noises and lights that make me dizzy. My mom took me to the car where I fell asleep. Missed the fireworks. Not a very exciting Fourth of July for me, but I needed the rest, my body was getting too low, and for me that can be dangerous.

I Get Tired   July 13, 2011

The doctor said that food wouldn't matter while I am on the Prednisone, but it does. We have come to notice that when I eat things that I was previously avoiding I get tired the way I did in Steamboat. My bowels are not directly affected because of the high doses of steroids, but my body is still not handling the food well. So, we have decided to try and watch what I eat more carefully and avoid things like gluten and dairy more often.

Today was another interesting appointment. Like I mentioned before, the prednisone can cause all kinds of crazy things to happen and one of the things is that it can make your bones really weak. Since I have been on the prednisone for a while now, my doctor called in a test called a "DexaScan", which is basically just a bone scan. I went in to have this scan done today to check that my bones are not being weakened to a dangerous point. All I did was lay under an x-ray type machine for a few minutes while they checked my bone density. All seems to be okay and my bones are nice and healthy.

Eye Doctor   *July 15, 2011*

Along with the "DexaScan" I have to have an "eye checkup" because surprise, surprise, steroids can mess up your eyes too… so we have to make sure that it isn't.

I went in to the eye doctor hoping that this would just be an easy check up where I read the wall and then get to go. But I was wrong.

This doctor was a nut job. He was super giddy and excited about everything; he actually kind of creeped me out. The whole reason that I went to this doctor was to see if I have too much pressure in my eyes from the medicine. So, as expected I had to read the wall, but that was not all I had to do. The doctor got out this little stick with a soft end and he said "Okay now just look ahead." Then, POKE! It felt like he poked my eye with the stick! Ouch, it hurt. Then he says, "Okay I won't do that again but now I just have to put a little puff of air in your eye." I thought, *"Whatever dude, do whatever you want, since you already poked my eye without telling me."* So, he got this little canister of air and "puffed" it into my eye. This was a strong puff, kind of like comparing a garden hose to a fire hose. Ouch! The good news is, my eyes are fine. But after all of that who knows, maybe now they have a problem from being poked and puffed.

I get to wear funny glasses the rest of the day to protect my eyes from light, what an interesting appointment that was.

Volleyball Camp
July 29, 2011

I have been at camp for a few days now but today is a funny day! The camp I am at is at Santa Clara University. A bunch of volleyball players come to this camp during the summer to train. We all get to say in the college dorms together and we wake up at 7AM to play volleyball and we play until 9 at night! (With breaks for food of course).

But anyway, today is a funny day because throughout the week I have been eating the dorm food because that is what we are provided with and since I am on the prednisone it shouldn't matter. I still avoid the real obvious gut bombs, like Mexican food for example. Last night we all went to the cafeteria for dinner and the hot meal happened to be, Mexican! I chose not to eat it and to have a salad instead, but most of the girls did eat the burritos. This morning when we woke up there was a huge line outside of the bathroom because the Mexican food hadn't sat well for anyone – if you know what I mean. Laughing at the whole situation I just found it all to be so funny, because usually that's me running for the bathroom but today, it was everyone else!

Last night was pretty funny too, because right before bed, before anyone knew that they would be sick in the morning, we spent an hour outside in our pajamas because someone had set off the fire alarm! I love this camp!

Kayaking Trip   August 13 and 14, 2011

I didn't bring my journal with me on the kayaking trip because I didn't want it to get wet, so I will write about it now that we are home.

The last two days my mom, my sister, my mom's friend, her two daughters and I all went kayaking together. We took the kayaks out to this little island and set up a campsite there. The weekend was spent swimming, kayaking, laughing and enjoying the lake! It was a wonderful girls weekend.

One of the days, my sister, and our two friends decided to go for a trip on the life raft that we had. We floated on it for hours, until we found ourselves in the middle of the lake! After hanging out on the raft, tanning and telling stories we all realized that we had to poop... All of us had to go. Unsure of what to do, because we were so far out an it would take at least an hour to get back to land, we saw a rock sticking out of the water. Paddling, we made it to the rock and stopped our boat. This rock was hardly big enough for one person to stand on, but it was enough to hold the raft still and that was all we needed. We all pulled our bikinis down and hung our bare bottoms off the side of the life raft and pooped. Anyone from a clear distance could see our bottoms hanging off the raft, but we didn't care, we had to go!

Everyone's poop did something different than mine, mine floated while theirs sunk. Now thank goodness that I am having somewhat normal poops right now because if I had exploded bloody diarrhea into the lake that would be whole other story!

Back To School

August 18, 2011

Today was the first day of school. Jeff is now dating someone else. I'm sad... but I know I don't need a boyfriend right now anyway. I have plenty of other things going on in my life, no need to complicate things more.

We are also starting to taper me off the Prednisone, so soon my puffiness along with my other side effects should be gone!

Here We Go Again   *August 20, 2011*

My mommy talked to doctor yesterday. It seems like things are starting to go bad again…

The doctor recommended that I start taking "Turmeric" supplements. Apparently this is an Indian spice that is known to help decrease inflammation. And they are hoping that this spice will help to bring down the inflammation I have in my colon right now. We'll see what happens!

Not Going Well

August 22, 2011

My taper from prednisone is not going well and I am "flaring". We started the turmeric like the doctor said and that seems to be making things worse, and fast! A few days ago I was just bleeding a little but now since we started the turmeric it has gone to being explosive, bloody diarrhea! What is going on?!

My mom called the doctor again to see what we should do. He said to stop the turmeric (that didn't last long) and increase the prednisone again. We need to get started on the next medication, but he wants to talk with us first.

Nobody knows what to do or why I am getting worse with everything we try. Right now we are just at a stand still until someone can figure something out.

My Birthday!   August 27, 2011

This birthday was much better than the last, no crazy thoughts or crying! But not perfect either. I think my birthday might be cursed. My disease seems to really like to show itself around my birthday every year. The taper from the prednisone isn't going so well. I am starting to flare up again and I have hemorrhoids galore!

For my birthday I got a brand new bike! One I had been wanting; I am so excited to have gotten it! We went for a short ride, but hemorrhoids and bikes aren't exactly friends. Not only do I have hemorrhoids, I also have actual burns around my rectum. They itch and burn so bad! I have been bleeding a little bit today but not too bad, things seem to be going back to the path we have been on before...

For my birthday meal we had:

> Spaghetti Bolognese, gluten free (brown rice noodles)
> Steamed broccoli
> Gluten free chocolate cake
> Watermelon

For the most part my birthday was great! Yummy cake, super dinner, great gifts, loving friends and family and much better than last year ☺

Things will get better; I have no complaints!

Long Talk   *August 28, 2011*

My mom has been researching the role of Salicylate Intolerance. She is starting to think that maybe that is why I can't handle the mesalamine medications.

We have so many questions, but nobody seems to have any answers...

> Why did the sulfasalazine work, but the other mesalamines didn't?
> Why didn't the dietary restrictions work the way we were told they would?
> Why did Turmeric just make my body freak-out?

As of right now I am no longer having the sad thoughts the way I was before. Ever since we stopped the Sulfasalazine I have been feeling fine, emotionally that is.

But today that wasn't the case, I was sad today.

I am sad because I am scared and frustrated with this disease. I still have the burns on my bottom from all the diarrhea I have been having. Basically my diarrhea has been so acidic that it has been burning off the skin on my bottom.

My mom and I had a long talk today. She explained what she has been reading and learning. She learned that foods high in Salicylate are linked to behavioral problems, mood swings, headaches and in some not so common instances... digestive problems. There are even a few reports of Ulcerative Colitis. She learned about an enzyme called Diamine Oxidase, which is supposed to help break down histamine in the gut. We don't really understand all of this, but for now we are going to try and restrict foods that contain high levels of salicylate. Nothing else has seemed to work....
Maybe this is worth a try.

Hair Analysis   *September 1, 2011*

I went to my local doctor for a hair analysis today. It didn't take long. All he did was lift up my hair grab a huge chunk from the right side and cut it, and then did the same on the left...

I can't put my hair in a ponytail without being able to see two funny little stubs of hair about a centimeter long. That's going to be weird when it starts to grow out...

Perfect! For volleyball season, I will look real funny because my hair has to be up. What is a girl to do?

Low Salicylate Diet   September 3, 2011

Right now I am still on the Prednisone. I am doing a little bit better than I was before, but not great. I still have pain and bloody diarrhea but it has gone down to about 5 times a day.

We are going to start a Low Salicylate Diet. We don't know much about this theory but are willing to give it a try. Yippee!!! This means I get a new food list! This is the list of food that I <u>can</u> eat!

<u>Any type of fresh meat – baked or grilled</u>
beef, chicken, turkey, pork, white fish – eggs also allowed
NO deli meats – contain nitrites and spices

<u>Grains</u>
wheat, rye, barley, oats, rice, amaranth

<u>Dairy</u>
butter, whole cream, lactose free milk, plain yogurt, white cheese (no blue or molded), sour cream

<u>Nuts</u>
cashews, hazelnuts, pecans, sunflower seeds

<u>Beans</u>
all beans (except Broad Beans and Fava Beans)
bean sprouts, lentils, chickpeas

<u>Fruits</u>
banana, golden delicious apple (peeled), lemon, lime, papaya, pomegranate, canned pears (peeled)

<u>Vegetables</u>
brussel sprouts, cabbage, cauliflower, peas, leek, onions, shallots, celery, iceberg lettuce, fresh mushrooms, old peeled white potato

<u>Spices</u>
salt, chives, fennel, garlic, parsley, saffron

<u>Oils</u>
sunflower, safflower, canola, butter

<u>Sweets</u>
white sugar, brown sugar, pure maple syrup, chocolate (no additives)

Yippee!! Chocolate…I LOVE chocolate! This is already my favorite diet so far!

Already Feeling Better! September 6, 2011

I am already feeling better! One big healthy looking poop this morning, that made my whole day!

We had a doctor appointment today.

The doctors want me to begin a medication called "6-MP" in combination with the prednisone AGAIN. This seems like such a big step. I am already improving with the change in diet and the 6MP raises so many worries about serious possible side effects. Not side effects like leg cramps but dangerous side effects. 6-MP is a form of chemotherapy medication and is a very powerful drug. To me this should be the very last resort because of all the dangers and I am not ready to give up on what we are trying just yet. Also, the reality of using a medication that would really suppress my immune system is scary. We have not had good results with medications so far, and we are not sure this would be the right course for me, especially since a relatively low percentage of people with Ulcerative Colitis actually seem to do well on 6-MP.

My mom asked the doctor if we could try to taper the prednisone again but this time I would be on the low salicylate dietary restrictions. Right now I am following the "Feingold List of Foods". These are foods that are low in salicylates and I am only allowed to have those that range from negligible to low in salicylates.

Hopefully the prednisone will have brought down the inflammation and the diet will keep it from getting inflamed again. That's the hope!

The doctor said that he had never heard of this and did not think it was possible. He then went on to tell us that he would be willing to allow a four-week evaluation of this dietary approach as long as we agreed to call if any problems occurred and also agreed to have colonoscopy after the four weeks.

We agreed! Fingers crossed, I hope this works!

Volleyball Day

September 10, 2011

I have been doing great! I am still taking probiotics and sticking to the diet, which seems to be working! Poop is good but today I had a terrible headache.

I was at a volleyball tournament all day with my team and it was raining super hard. Each team had a tent set up outside the gym and that is where we waited for our match to start and where we ate our lunch. It was cold and raining but the moms had set out a wonderful array of sandwich making supplies under our tent. I made myself a sandwich by putting turkey on tortilla.

A few hours after lunch I got a TERRIBLE HEADACHE and could barely play... I felt so awful. When the tournament was over I just slept the whole way home.

I wonder why I got that headache?

Yuck   *September 11, 2011*

Yucky! The entire sandwich from yesterday seems to have passed straight through me without being digested at all.

Apparently my body did not like it too much.

After that experience, my mom and I decided no more deli meat or heavily processed breads for a while.

High Levels Of Bismuth? September 13, 2011

My hair samples came back and tested really high for Bismuth. Nobody knows what that means. Somehow Bismuth binds with salicylates, but I'm not really sure how this works. But I do know that adds some hope to our Low Salicylate Diet!

Do You Like Rice?   September 22, 2011

I have been following my dietary rules of only eating low salicylate content foods. I'm off the prednisone and all is good! Everything seems to be normal for a change, What a relief that is!

Kids at school know that I have a disease now because I had to tell them why I eat weird food. They think I just get a little tummy ache when I eat the wrong food, and that is all I want them to think.

But at school today, this boy in my class really pissed me off. I was in the cafeteria, minding my own business, just waiting for the microwave so I could heat up my, rice. Yes, shocker, rice. I have been eating rice for weeks and don't mind it. I actually do like rice. But I didn't like it when this rude boy came up to me and said, "All you eat is rice, do you really like rice or something?"

...Yeah, bingo... I have a creepy addiction to rice and that is why I eat rice all day long. I actually eat it for breakfast and dinner too... Plain white rice, all day, yummy! He wasn't trying to be rude. His comment just annoyed me. I mean honestly, does he really think that I just like rice soooo much that I eat it every day. No! Who would do that for fun!? He knows I have a disease and that is why I eat funny, I mean seriously, did he really feel the need to ask me that when he already knew the answer...

To add to my frustration, the cutest boy in school is still dating that other girl. They are lasting longer than I thought they would. Bummer. Otherwise, life is great!

Things Are Changing Again
October 19, 2011

This evening I had what I like to call "sludge-poop". It's not formed or diarrhea, its just kind of this nasty sludge that just seeps out of me. Nasty, I know. But what changed?

All was good up until now...

Yesterday my coach was yelling at volleyball, so that was kind of stressful; and I had another deli sandwich with ham and turkey... maybe not the best idea...

Being Careful *October 22, 2011*

Over the last few weeks I have come to notice that whenever I eat gluten and dairy I have some sort of a reaction, whether that be a severe headache, a stomach ache, nausea, a stuffy nose or some bleeding. So we have decided that maybe my body is not ready to start digesting gluten and dairy since both are difficult to digest anyway. As of now I am being more careful with gluten and dairy since I never feel good after having bread or milk.

I have my colonoscopy coming up soon anyway, so that will help us to know what is really going on in my colon and see if we have made any improvement from the time that I had my last colonoscopy.

Colonoscopy Today!   October 27, 2011

Yippee! Today is the day where I get to go to the hospital, lay in a gown, and have a team of nurses crowd around my butt while a doctor sticks a camera up it and takes a look around. How exciting!

But strangely enough, I actually am excited. I am kind of looking forward to the results of this colonoscopy. The last one was not so great, things were looking rough inside, but I think things have gotten better since then and I am curious what my colon looks like. Strange, I know, but I'm interested.

Although I am excited for the results, I am not excited for the procedure. Last night I drank 2 gallons of "Go Lightly" (colonoscopy prep) which tastes worse than horse pee. It burns the whole way down. I can feel it from the moment I swallow till the moment I poop it out. The way "Go Lightly" works is that it cleans you out so the doctor has a clear view when the camera goes inside. So, I had to drink, drink, drink, drink until I was literally peeing clear liquid out of my butt. It was wonderful. Not exactly how I wanted to spend my afternoon, but hey, as long as you aren't more that 30 feet from the toilet, all is good.

Today, I am starving and just can't wait to fall asleep so that when I wake up I can eat again. I see popsicles in my near future!

Just to add to the discomfort of a colonoscopy, I am also on my period, which makes the whole procedure just that much more disgusting!

++++++++++

I'm awake now and feeling great, well for having just been under anesthesia that is. I am still a little drowsy but I'm starting to come to now.

I have good news!

The doctors were baffled when they saw my test results. They said they had never seen anything like it and the fact that I am doing this well without any medicine is near impossible. My colon looks great and shows good evidence of healing!
Halleluiah!

Gluten Free Isn't So Bad   November 4, 2011

Yesterday me, my mommy and sister decided to make gluten free donuts since I have been craving a Crispy Cream for days and homemade gluten free is as close as we are going to get. They were surprisingly delicious! We made them using brown rice and sorghum flour and then coated them (heavily) in powdered sugar.

Actually, they were so good that I ate twelve! Today I am starting to rethink if that was such a good idea… Let's just say that they were yummy on the way in, but not so yummy on the way out…I have horrible deadly gas.

Thanksgiving in Colorado   *November 24, 2011*

This time, we are in Colorado because the whole family is getting together for Thanksgiving! There will be about 40 people in my Aunt's tiny house, but this get together is always a blast!
With my family, nothing is boring.

Surprisingly enough, my dinner wasn't all that boring either, I mean compared to everyone else's. Clearly I cannot enjoy the pumpkin pie, mashed potatoes, stuffing or glazed turkey considering I can't eat any spices, milk or gluten... This didn't really matter, because my mommy made a fantastic "Heather Dinner" for me with all the food that I am allowed. The funny thing was that, everyone really liked my food and actually preferred it to some of the other dishes.
I'm feeling great!

I am thankful for my health right now, my family for their support and life for pushing me just hard enough that I can grow stronger but never break.

Uh Oh...
November 27, 2011

I get this feeling sometimes that I like to call "Jiminy Cricket." The reason I call this sensation that is because that is how it feels. When I first described the feeling I said that "I feel like there is a little "Jiminy Cricket" marching around in my colon." It doesn't hurt, or cause any sort of pain, just a feeling, like tapping from the inside of my colon. Like that little cricket is in there stomping around.

Overall, I'm not feeling very good. I know that when I have "Jiminy Cricket" that it is not a good thing, because I shouldn't be having these feelings. At first, I thought these feelings were good, and that I was feeling my colon heal. But now, I have come to learn that when I start to feel this, bad things tend to follow.

And I was right. We flew home from Colorado yesterday and the only food that there was available was what we could find in or near the airport. Which is not the kind of food my body is used to eating. Since things had gone so well while we were on vacation, my family as a whole, thought that one night out for dinner couldn't hurt... but we were wrong, because today I have "Jiminy Cricket" and a yucky feeling inside.

Food is definitely an issue for me. Now I know, that just because I am feeling good does not mean that I can break away from the rules, I have to stick with this!

At The Doctor All The Time...   December 6, 2011

Another doctors appointment! I feel like I am in this waiting room with this hyper nurse far too often! But hopefully I won't have to come back for a while, since today the doctor told me that things are sounding good and that whatever it is we are doing seems to be working. All has been going well so far. I mean, there are a few days here and there of odd poop, but otherwise good. But really... Who doesn't have funny poops sometimes... its not like normal people just poop exactly the same every time they go... right?

Yank...   *December 7, 2011*

I had my wisdom teeth pulled out today... Not a flattering experience. I went in to the office, bright and early this morning, sat in a chair and had some laughing gas. All went well. Until, I woke up. It hurt so badly! Not only did I wake up in pain, I was confused. I was sure I was in a closet... Strange thing is I didn't have a sweatshirt on before I went into surgery, but when I woke up I was wearing one. Strange. Who put that on me?

Tonight was also my volleyball banquet for the end of season and awards. I had to be there.

Earlier, I couldn't feel my face. I had a freak out and started crying because I thought that the doctor had cut off my tongue; I honestly could not feel it in my mouth. Then I spent the rest of the afternoon drooling on myself and spilling applesauce down my chin. To add to my attractiveness I had an ace bandage tied like a bow around my head, holding two ice packs on either cheek. Getting one tooth pulled hurts... getting four pulled; that REALLY hurts.

SO, anyway, back to volleyball. I had to go to this banquet. So, I put some makeup on my very rounded face and went with the plan of sitting quietly in the back. But, the coach called my name to come up and receive an award! He tried to talk with me in front of everyone, but my mouth was still numb, so I just made mumbling sounds and drooled. So embarrassing! To make matters even worse, he gave me a big old pat on the back, which rattled things around a bit and made my teeth hurt and even bleed a little.

I should not have gone to the banquet!

Mucus Everywhere!   December 12, 2011

My wisdom teeth didn't heal quite right. I had something called an "impacted extraction." I thought the tooth extraction hurt, but I had no idea how much worse the impaction hurts! Maybe I should have stayed home instead of going back to school so soon.

Today, I had to go back to the doctor. He basically soaked a cotton ball in some medicine and stuck it in the hole where my tooth had once been. Ouch!

Some days I think my body hates me. On top of the wisdom tooth problem, I also have a sinus infection and have been blowing my nose all day long! Thing is that not only do I have mucus in my nose, it is also in my poop. I have been having some mucus discharge and a little bit of blood in my poop. I don't get as scared about this as I used to. Besides, the diamond in the rough is that I am only going about one to two times per day!

Saxophone Christmas   December 17, 2011

We are in the bay area this weekend for *Saxophone Christmas* where like 200 saxophone players all get together early in the morning and practice a bunch of Christmas songs together. Then in the afternoon they have a huge performance in the park. The whole thing is just amazing!

My dad and sister both played in it today and did great. As they were off practicing their music, my mom and I got to sleep in at the hotel and enjoy a morning of rest. After a sleep in, we went down to the hotel breakfast bar to get some food. Thinking ahead, my mom had brought some eggs with us so that I could eat them for breakfast; she even had them pre-boiled! What we didn't think about was that the eggs were cold, since we had kept them in the fridge in the room. Now, I don't know how most people eat their eggs, but I like mine hot!

So, I put one egg on a plate and into the microwave – just for a few seconds. When the egg was nice and warm, I took it out and was ready to eat! Just as I was about to bite into it, my mom suggested that we cut it into smaller pieces. The moment the knife touched the egg; the egg exploded! It literally sounded like a bomb. Egg went everywhere; in my hair, all over the plate and on both of our faces! The whole restaurant turned to look at what we had done; probably scared we were terrorists coming to bomb the place with our egg bombs.

All I can say is thank goodness I didn't bite into that egg, because then, the explosion would have been in my mouth. And, from this… we have learned not to microwave boiled eggs!

Tahoe Trip
December 20, 2011

We have been skiing at Tahoe again with our friends, but all day today I had severe pain in my belly button. Turning, bending and even walking would send a shooting pain through my belly button and all around my stomach. Given the circumstances of my disease I got pretty freaked out. This intense pain started to make me nervous, so my mom and I went back to the house we are renting to take a break. When the rest of the group came in from the day of skiing the pain was still there. It was starting to feel like someone was stabbing a needle into my belly button over and over, every time I moved.

After much debate and the pain increasing, we headed to the emergency room at Tahoe and sat in the car in the parking lot. None of us knew what to do. Stomach pain in someone with Ulcerative Colitis is probably a bad thing. What if the doctor wanted to admit me? What if there were going to be more tests? I couldn't even think about being in a strange hospital.

I found that when I pushed on my belly button the pain got increasingly worse. This didn't seem like the pain or Jiminy Crickets I sometimes have in my stomach. Unsure about what to do, we called my aunt and told her what was going on. I really don't know why we called her, but we did. She thought maybe my abdominals were sore from skiing. I had a bad fall yesterday. She assured us that muscle pain increases when pressure is applied and that if it were something wrong with my stomach, pushing on it would make it feel better.

Deciding that this was probably just a muscle ache since this was the first real ski day of the season and my body was weak, we went back to the house. Sure enough, the pain went away a few hours later. It was just a scare. But with a history of having holes in my intestines and bleeding out of my butt, a stomach ache can be pretty nerve racking.

A White Christmas

December 25, 2011

This Christmas was a white one! We woke up to a snow covered deck and the sun just beginning to rise over the valley. It was magnificent! A truly white Christmas!

Gifts, dairy free hot chocolate, family, friends, love and Christmas cheer was all around us today. We exchanged the many holiday surprises we had gotten for each other; all which were perfect! My mommy and papa even surprised us with a foosball table to go in the basement. The rest of our day was spent at home relaxing and enjoying the beautiful holiday.

Following tradition, we made a superb Christmas feast and spent the rest of the night together. This Christmas was great! We are really starting to get a hang of cooking, so dinner was even more delicious than last year!

Pork tenderloin
String beans with cashews
Buttered potatoes mashed with hemp milk
Gluten free chocolate cake with lemon sorbet

After dinner and desert, we had an intense foosball tournament in the basement! Papa won...

Another Hair Analysis?! *January 18, 2012*

Once again, the time has come for the doctor to lift my luscious locks and chop off a significant chunk of them. This really is not something I enjoy. I do not like having centimeter length hair sticking away from my neck at the base of my head. Well, it is only noticeable when I wear my hair up, which I do quite frequently. So, it is therefore noticeable. But that's not the worst part! The worst part, by far, is when the hair starts to grow, but it's not long enough to fit in any sort of up-do. It just hangs there awkwardly. It is an inconvenient, awkward, 2-inch long chunk of hair. Last time, I attempted pinning it up, but the hair was so short that the chunk would slip out of the pins and just hang on the side of my head. It's awful! I'm just going to have to get used to wearing my hair down for a while so people can't really see the nub.

It's kind of embarrassing. People probably think I'm some sort of alien that has to be genetically tested all the time and that's why I have funny hairs stick out of my ponytail. If only that were the case… The reality is, I am a sick child and nobody can really tell me why.

Is Sausage A No-Go? *January 22, 2012*

Yesterday I scarfed down a delicious chicken and apple sausage. I have been on the diet for five months now and things seem to be improving and then getting worse again… It's a constant rollercoaster with this disease. One day I am healthy, the next I am sick. What is going on in my body?! How much longer will I be on this diet… and how do we even know if it is working if all that happens is, I get sick and then I get better, then get sick, then get better…

Today is one of those not-so-good days…

I woke up running to the bathroom, which is something I am very familiar with. Then, when I looked to see what I had pooped out today, I saw mucus and lots of it. There hasn't been blood in a while, which is good. But mucus is not much better. When there is mucus in my stool, it means my colon in inflamed and producing mucus, which it then gets rid of through my poop. This is not the same mucus as when you blow your nose. The mucus I see in the toilet looks like little white worms, swimming all around the toilet bowl and then at the bottom is a pile of sludge, not poop, yellowish-brown sludge.

My hair analysis came back today as well… no change. Exactly the same results as last time. Chunks of hair growing out the sides of my neck, but nothing new learned… what now?

Never-ending Medical Case   January 31, 2012

I feel like a never-ending medical case!

It seems like nobody on this planet can tell me *why* I have this disease or how to make it go away. We don't have a family history, I never drank dirty water in some third world country, I was only on antibiotics once when I was a kid, and we eat healthy. My eighth grade year at school was pretty stressful, but is that enough?

Then today I go and mess up my leg on the slopes and have to go to the Ski Patrol room to have it fixed up. At least someone can tell me exactly what I did to my knee and exactly how to fix it. Let me tell you, that is a refreshing change. The ski patrol visit was the first "doctor's visit" I have left free of questions in the last two and a half years!

Ski patrol explained that my kneecap is just the slightest bit off center and when I went to tear up some moguls this morning I over-exerted one of my muscles and caused it to give out on me. This resulted in a fall, which resulted in an extremely painful knee, which brought me to the Ski Patrol office where I laid on a table having my knee iced and massaged. It was a nice bit of TLC!

Strangely enough I actually enjoyed this little accident. I liked going to see the "doctor" and having him know what was wrong. When something like Ulcerative Colitis leaves so many questions in my life, the appreciation of an answer goes up significantly.

Since I have a cold, again, I chose to stay in the rest of the day and keep off my knee the way the Ski Patrol had told me. I feel like I am always sick with a cold. No matter what, I have a stuffy nose and don't feel so great. Because I feel like this so much of the time, I have come to be used to it and just kind of consider it normal, but it is not. Maybe this has something to do with my disease. I have noticed that when I have a flare, my cold symptoms get significantly worse too... And today I feel my cold getting worse, does that mean I will be sick soon?

Warning Signs

February 1, 2012

The never-ending cold must be related, because this morning I woke up with "fuzzy poop". This may sound strange, but I do not know how else to describe it. There is a normal-ish looking poop but then all around it is white fuzz. I don't know why or how that even happens, but it did and my cold is worse today too… Everything seems to be connected.

I'm not feeling well and my fuzzy poop came about 4 times today, urgently. I still went skiing, but no worries, my knee was all taped up and stabilized. Everything was great except for the fact that I wanted to be enjoying my wonderful ski day a lot more than I was. But how happy can one be when there is a constant worry? The answer is: not so happy… today.

I just don't understand. I stick to my diet, ALWAYS! I take all the probiotics and supplements that we have been told to use. Why doesn't this disease just leave me alone?

Eggs   *February 18, 2012*

So, ever since the day of the fuzzy poop, I have been feeling just fine. All is good, but I have realized that

> *I just don't like eggs.*

Every time I eat eggs I don't feel good. I get irritable and cranky, have a pounding headache and I feel way more exhausted than normal. Eggs do something funky to me...

Another thing I have noticed is that whenever I eat eggs my scary thoughts come back. It's a strange relationship, but eggs bring back my sad thoughts. I am sure of it. Also, they make me crazy! I freak out about everything and cry all the time...

Eggs just don't seem like something I should be eating right now; so I'm not going to eat them! As yummy as I think they are, and as good for you as they are, I don't think eggs are a good thing for **My** body. Not because they make my disease flare, but because they make my head hurt and I feel crazy!

I am actually kind of scared of eggs. That sounds nuts, but I actually think I might have a legitimate fear of eggs. They scare me. I don't like the idea that something I eat can make my crazies come back.

I think I am an "Ovophobic." But, maybe that's not so bad. Did you know Alfred Hitchcock had a fear of eggs?

At least I'm not the only one.

That is something that I think is really important to remember throughout this whole experience. Although nobody can truly understand how I feel or what I am going through; I am not the only one. Everyone faces their own battles. No battle is larger or more important than another. I know that nothing is impossible. I can over come this because *I'm*Possible.

Fingers Crossed

February 27, 2012

Today I went in for the IgG food testing blood labs. Just like last time (about a year ago), my blood was sent off to Florida! The results should come back in a few weeks. We are really hoping for different results than last time. This would be nice not only because it would provide me with more food options but also because that would show that I am healing and that maybe I react to fewer foods now… Fingers crossed!

Changing diets and avoiding certain foods all the time can be so tiring. Once in a while I just so desperately want to go out for dinner with friends and not be the awkward one at the table that has to ask the waitress a million questions before I can order. The waitresses always seem to get a little annoyed; like I'm that obnoxious picky girl that doesn't want to eat too many carbs… But in reality, I would love to just eat something off any ol' menu at any restaurant.

Results Are In — March 13, 2012

The IgG test results came back today. My mom and I saw the letter in the stack of mail. We saw the letterhead from the lab in Florida and knew that my results were inside. Holding the letter, we were nervous to open it. The list inside this letter would determine my menu for God knows how long... Maybe avoiding foods high in salicylates has helped my colon heal. But then again, what if nothing had changed? What if I had spent all of this time eating so carefully to find out that I still have a leaky gut?

Nervous, we opened it and read the results aloud. Most things remain the same as last time, but it seems like the list just got longer. I have antibodies against:

- Baker's Yeast
- Beef
- Brewer's yeast
- Egg
- Milk
- Mustard
- Peanut
- Soybean
- Wheat
- Green Peas
- Lamb
- Peach
- Pinto Beans
- Benzoic Acid – preservative
- Gluten
- Hazelnut

Brewers yeast was one that stood out to me... I have never even had a beer. In elementary school, I was never really introduced to alcohol and grew up a very innocent child. Then, obviously, in high school I was not able to drink because of my disease. Not only have I not had alcohol because of the food restrictions but because I am terrified of not having control. This whole experience has opened my eyes to so many new things.

When I was diagnosed, I had no control over what happened to me. I got sick and my life changed forever and I had no say in that. I did not ask for this to happen to me nor did I want it. This disease has affected my views on life though... I can't watch other people throw their health away without it hurting me. Now, my friends go out and party and have a few drinks once in a while. That does not bother me. But the kids who are avid drinkers and who use tobacco products daily or use other drugs; watching them actually hurts me. They don't know how fortunate they are to have a normally functioning body. But what can I say? They won't care what I think, I am just that "good girl" who thinks drugs are bad. That isn't true. Yes, I don't agree with drugs and overconsumption of alcohol, but that is not because I think they are bad. It is because I have come to appreciate life and health so much more since my diagnosis, that when I see others throwing away the good thing that they have, I can't bear to watch. I don't expect them to understand, because before I was sick I never really appreciated being healthy, so why would they even think about it. You truly don't know what you have until its gone...

++++++++++

Anyway... back to the food sensitivity list.
Hmmm... what to do with this? The list is just as long as before with only a few new changes. Yet, this list does not have the same sensitivities as the Salicylate list does. So, which one do I follow? Which list has the real foods that I am sensitive to? Do I not eat Salicylates or do I follow this new list? I'm confused but I guess we are going to start following this list for now and see what happens, then we will go from there.

I won't miss the egg or milk; so that's good! My fear of eggs won't be getting in the way of this diet and hopefully by cutting eggs out completely then no more sad thoughts. They still come and go occasionally but for the most part they are much better; except for when I eat eggs. But since this new diet eliminates eggs, it should eliminate that problem as well!

We have decided to stick with a rotation for the wheat/gluten. The new IgG list says NO WHEAT but the Salicylate list says that wheat is okay... and since I am in desperate need for some bread, we have decided to have a "bread day". Bread day is going to be AMAZING! I get to eat a little bit of bread once a week. This may sound like nothing but when you haven't eaten bread in a year and you crave bread and butter on a daily basis; one slice of bread is like heaven, even if it is only once a week!

My mommy also called the doctor that did IgG test today. He told her that after a few weeks it would be okay to SLOWLY add food back into my diet that are not on this list. He doesn't think the salicylate list is as important anymore. Mommy and I talked about this and decided that the first thing we want to start adding back in slowly would be some fruits. Adding fruit to my diet would make eating on the go MUCH easier!

Apparently I Stink Up The Bus...   *March 10, 2012*

I hate having to pack all of my own food for tennis. It's embarrassing! In route to every away game we stop at the gas station to get lunch. Everyone else on the team gets a burrito or a sandwich, a soda or even a slushy and I sit in the car with my lunch box and its strange contents. Sometimes I can't even eat my lunch; it tastes so bad. With what she has to work with, my mom does an amazing job! And everyday she is getting better at making yummy food! But every once in a while there is a tester meal that just doesn't work out. When gluten free, dairy free, taste free food doesn't work out…it's gross!

The worst part about eating my lunch on the tennis bus is that it usually smells kind of funny… As soon as I open my Tupperware I hear the back seat whining, every time… "that's gross" "that smells disgusting" "roll the window down" "I'm going to be sick; eat that later."

I hate those comments. I'm just as hungry as you are and you don't see me complaining about your nasty bagged burrito stinking up the whole bus. SO, let me eat my gluten free pasta with funny beef and vegetables in peace. People make me so angry. They know I have a reason to be eating this kind of food. Obviously this isn't by choice, so leave me alone about it. Sometimes, I am just as unhappy about eating it as you are smelling it, but you don't see me complaining… Ugg some people…

I'm Feeling Good!!!   *March 26, 2012*

Today is a good day! I haven't been writing in my journal as much lately because when I am doing good I have less reason to write. This is my place to let out my thoughts and my feelings. When I am hurt or sick it helps me to release my anger and fears onto paper instead of onto others. Although I know I am not alone on this journey, I do not want to burden others with the constant stress and worries that are along this road. I don't want to worry them too much, so I write here.

The fact that I haven't written in a while is a good thing! All is good ☺

I Cheated...   *March 28, 2012*

There was blood today… Not a lot. Just a little. But I think I know why.

I cheated. I have never really cheated before but I did this weekend. All weekend I was away at a volleyball tournament and there was food everywhere! Our team went out for dinner one night at a Chinese restaurant, and I ate. I had some chicken and some rice thinking that would be safest, but I should have known better. Asian food has so many spices and sauces and well, to be honest, I don't really know what they put in their food… But now, I know that whatever it is, my body doesn't like it. Silly Heather… at least we know now; Chinese food is a negative!

But really, I can't cheat off my diet one time! One time! It's like I am being punished or something… Ugg… How much longer?! Will it ever end?!

Playing With Monkeys   April 4-7, 2012

I forgot to bring my journal with me on my trip so I have to remember about it now that I am back. Over this spring break, my mommy, my sister and I all went to Shreveport, Louisiana to visit one of my mom's old college friends!

This was not just an ordinary visit. Her friend helps to run Chimp Haven, a sanctuary for chimpanzees that used to be used for drug testing and other science experiments. They are rescue chimps and there are hundreds of them. The facility is set up so that there is an indoor enclosure and an outdoor one. The outdoor enclosure is not really an enclosure though, it is the wilderness, and just how the animals would live out in nature. Given acres and acres of land to roam the chimpanzees are happy there. They socialize, they are well fed, taken care of and they are living happily away from the cages and science experiments they were exposed to before.

At this incredible place we got to visit some of the chimps. We talked to them and threw toys for them. Watched a mama and her baby climb a tree and we even had a chimp spit on us! When my sister and I were walking past one of the enclosures a chimpanzee came running up to the fence and spit right at my sister! It got all over her shirt and it was gross! Also the chimpanzees were really excited to have visitors. They are more humanlike than we realize! When we would walk through their enclosures they would wave at us and chirp. They screamed and screamed! When we walked by they would run in circles around big playgrounds and would run to the top to get a better look at us! We were so close to these animals, it was incredible. When you look into the eyes of a chimpanzee it is almost as though you can relate to them… they are so humanlike and they send off as certain aura… like they understand.

The trip to Shreveport was magnificent! And one of the best things about the trip was that my mommy was able to cook most of our meals at the house and I was safe on my diet the whole time!

Introducing Fruits　　　　　　*April 24, 2012*

So, we started introducing fruits back into my diet. But, maybe we jumped the gun…

We were so excited to have the opportunity to put a strawberry on my plate that I might have had too many.

Remembering that the doctors swore by the rotation in the past we are thinking that maybe we should use the rotation to help introduce new foods. My body needs to be introduced to the food but then be allowed a few days to welcome it back. Apparently, if I eat too many new things too fast, my body freaks out. I don't want to eat too much of a good thing, because I am really looking forward to fruit again.
Those strawberries were SO good!

PROM!   May 12, 2012

A senior asked me to prom!

The other day during tennis practice, some kids came up to the tennis courts and said they needed me to answer some questions about tennis for the yearbook. I followed them because they also said they needed a picture of me and that the picture had to be taken by the school sign. We walked down to the sign but on the way a bunch of boys popped out of the back of a red pick-up truck with a sign that read "PROM?" Then music started blasting from inside the truck and this guy I know who is a senior walked out from behind the truck! Clearly, I said yes and was super excited to be going to prom as a sophomore!

Tonight was the dance and it was amazing! I wore a beautiful turquoise, floor-length dress, studded with jewels. I felt like a princess. When he came to pick me up we took pictures of course, and my parents, being the funny joke-cracking people that they are did their best to embarrass me. But after living in this family for 15 years, I am invincible to embarrassment.

He took me in his truck to a friend's house, which had gorgeous tables set up across the expansive lawn. Each table had an elegant white cloth and flowers in the middle. Music played and dinner was served! I felt kind of out of place because I was the only sophomore at a party of seniors. Nobody was paying much attention to me, so I don't think they noticed that I barely ate. After dinner we all lined up on the grass where the parents had set up a little backdrop and some funny hats for us all to have a "group photo-shoot". This was really fun! The parents stood on the roof and took tons of pictures of us all posing with the set and all the fun hats. We even had big picture frames that we put our faces in to look like we were holding up a picture of us over our faces! The whole thing was just really cute! When everyone left and pulled out onto the road, our whole dinner party of about 10 cars decided to race to prom, which was about 10 miles away. We zoomed off in the red truck and laughed as we rolled down the windows. A red light ruined our chance of winning the race, but we were close!

The dance was beautiful, so much more elegant than any other high school dance. At the end of the night he tried to kiss me... But I looked away quickly. The boy was a sweetheart, and a good friend, but not someone I was attracted to… We had a really nice night together but that was all. I heard that Jeff and his girlfriend finally broke up; and the good news is, I am starting to talk to him again! They lasted about six months, longer than I expected, but all I care about is that she is gone and he is free! How could I kiss another guy at prom?

Cold Season   May 18, 2012

I don't know why I get a cold much more frequently than "every once in a while" or "during cold season." For me, every season is cold season! Yay for me! I have this chronic stuffy nose and it seems like I cough all the time. But the past few days it has gotten much worse. My cough went from being that dry little "cough, cough" that everyone gets sometimes to being the nasty wet cough that makes nobody want to be near you! It's icky. And when I cough it hurts! Just for a little icing on the cake, I also constantly have snot on my upper lip, because it drips out of my nose so frequently I can't always catch it with a tissue. Gross!

Last night my mom and I decided it was time for some cough syrup since my cough has been keeping the whole house up for days. We went to the doctor and she said it was just a virus – "should get better in a few days." I just don't know why they don't understand that when I get sick, I get really sick!

But, cough syrup has high fructose corn syrup in it. We have been told that high fructose corn syrup is bad for someone with a food intolerance to corn, but I needed to get some sleep! We thought, "one teaspoon of cough syrup couldn't do any harm." Wrong! I pooped blood and mucus this morning. But was it the cough syrup or was it that colitis can flare when the immune system is in high gear fighting another illness? Which is it? Even though we have told ourselves in the past that "one little bit can't hurt" it seems like a little bit seems to put my body over some kind of threshold.

Also, it is the end of the school year and we are having finals like crazy! My grades have slipped a little bit this semester because of all that I have been coping with from my disease. They haven't slipped much but I have a chance to get all my grades back to the normal "A" with my finals; so I have been studying like crazy! Of course, every doctor has told me that stress can make my disease flare. I don't know why this had to happen to me! After these finals I just need to relax and let my body rest for a few days! Hopefully then everything will be back to normal, including my grades!

Two Years   *June 15, 2012*

It has been two years since I found myself in that cold hospital room filled with uncertainty and fear. Seems that today deserves a journal entry.

I am still scared at times, but I have come a long way since that day... No, I am not completely healed. I still have good days and bad days, but mostly good days. Some days there is a little bit of blood on the tissue, some days a little bit of blood and mucus in my poop. Still, most days are good. I have come a long way. There is no longer a toilet filled with bloody sludge 10 or more times a day and I don't have to run to the bathroom anymore. I know that when I get "the feeling" I need to find a bathroom, but I don't need to run. The first year was hell! Compared to that, I am doing great. I am really aware of small changes and improvements in my disease. Even though it seems like this just happened overnight with no warning, I know that it is not something I can fix overnight.

I have been rotating fruits and that seems to be going all right. I think. At least I haven't had any severe reactions to the new introductions so I am pretty excited! Especially since it is summer, and who doesn't like a nice slice of watermelon or a strawberry by the pool! It's still, no wheat, no corn, no soy, no dairy, and no eggs for me! I don't miss the eggs or the dairy. That's easy. My mom has learned to bake with a "fake egg" that is flax seed, warm water and baking soda. We have found all kinds of non-dairy, nut based milks. But not eating wheat is still a bummer because wheat is delicious! Our rotation of the "bread-day" hasn't really worked out. I have a little bit every once in a while. Not much. Strange as this may seem, I miss soy the most! Not because I like tofu or soy sauce, but because soy is in everything! Soy lecithin is a main ingredient in all kinds of stuff, even gum! It's crazy. I will be in the grocery store and pick up something off the shelf, excited while I'm reading the ingredients, because it seems that everything in it is okay, and then I get to the very end and "soy lecithin" is there. Darn it! I can't even chew a stick of gum for goodness sake! That, I don't fully understand. I don't swallow gum... I don't digest the actual gum but, since there is soy in it, I am not allowed to have it. Also, gum is a no, no on the Salicylate list. I pretty much try to strictly avoid anything that falls on *both* the IgG list AND the Salicylate list. Crazy right?

It's not like I am starving or anything. In fact, I think my weight is perfect! Looking good and love to exercise. We make almost everything fresh ourselves. The best thing about the last few months is that my mom has become a better cook. She even bakes some killer gluten free, dairy free, egg free cookies!

Finally Mine! *June 20, 2012*

Today is a day I have been waiting for since the first day of math class, freshman year. The cutest boy in school is finally mine! For the last 2 weeks of sophomore year we have been partners in building a model home for our Geometry and Design class. Throughout this project he has spent a lot of time at my house building tiny houses out of styrofoam and we reconnected all over again. He would drive me to my house after school every day where we would build our houses and he would sing to me in the car on the way there. I laughed at how cute he was and knew that things were starting to fall back into place, right were they belonged; with me.

Today, he was over at my house. He was just about to leave and we were talking at the top of his driveway by his truck. In a few days he is going on a trip with his family and I won't see him for a couple of weeks. Then it happened! He kissed me and asked if I would finally be his girlfriend!

YES! Absolutely yes!

This is the moment I have been waiting for! I am finally dating the cutest boy in school… I knew he would come back for me; I knew he really cared!

Everything is perfect! I'm not bleeding when I poop and I have the most amazing guy to finally call mine!

Camp Counselor   *July 9, 2012*

This summer I started working at a children's summer camp in town. I am responsible for fifteen little 5 and 6 year olds! I really enjoy this camp and love playing and spending time with the kids. I think one of the reasons I really enjoy being with children is because they are so innocent and so happy. They have few worries and they can just run around and be happy. Their biggest fear is falling on the playground and they don't even really need to be afraid, because they know that I am there to catch them. We have water days where we set up a huge slip and slide and we play outside everyday! I love these kids! Each and every one of them is important to me. As fun as being a camp counselor is, it comes along with some difficult responsibilities. These kids trust me and want to tell me things; but sometimes hearing what they have to say can be hard. Hearing some of the things they tell me breaks my heart. I know that it is important to be there for them so that they have someone to talk to, someone they trust.

Fist Full Of Pills   July 20, 2012

Sometimes I feel like a drug addict! Even though I am not on any prescription medication right now I am really loading up on the supplements. Things like Aloe Vera to bring down the inflammation and VSL Probiotics to increase the amount of good buggies in my gut, folic acid since the foods that have folic acid aren't a part of my diet, vitamin C to help out my immune system, vitamin B for energy, and vitamin D3 to help… I don't really know what. Every morning I load up on these pills to help my body heal. When I go on trips I have to bring my pills with me, obviously, but the thing is, it is hard to transport them. My mom and I went to the pharmacy the other day to get a pillbox because I am going to spend some time on a houseboat with Jeff and the family of some other friends. I am so excited but I don't want to be a weirdo with plastic bags full of pills, so we went to find a case. Lucky me, all the cases were too small for my truck-load of pills… Not one pillbox we found would hold my daily handful! That's nuts! There is no way that I take more pills than everyone else! What about those old men on TV that complain about how many pills they have to take everyday… What kind of pillbox do they use, because I want one of those!

I was kind of embarrassed when we showed up to the house boat, because my mom, worried about me having enough to eat, practically packed the whole kitchen for one weekend. We had to load my two big bags of food and a cooler onto the boat. That's it; they have to think I'm a nut job by now… I lug around my whole kitchen and I eat out of my personal cooler. I must be crazy. My boyfriend didn't mind though and that's all that mattered to me. He knows everything and he doesn't judge one bit, he even carried all of my bags onto the boat for me. What a sweetheart! I'm a lucky girl. He actually likes the cookies my mom makes. Other than having to resort to my personal cooler and bags of food that I brought with me on this trip, the houseboat was amazing! We spent all day out on the water and played with jet skis and the boat, we went fishing and swimming and lay in the sun! It was a perfect little getaway and the first big thing I have done with my boyfriend!

Also something kind of embarrassing that has become a part of my life is calling to talk about food. Whenever I go to a restaurant I call ahead to ask about their menu. So, like that, my mommy called the dad of the kid whose houseboat we would be staying on this weekend to ask about what they had in mind for food. He told her they would be making chicken teriyaki (I can't eat the sauce) so they would leave the sauce off mine. My mom also told him that I couldn't eat any wheat and he responded by saying "No worries! We will pick up a nice white bread instead." I guess it is not easy for people to understand, but even good old-fashioned white bread is made with wheat! Oh well, it worked out. I just didn't eat any bread and hoped they didn't notice.

I Am Officially A Surfer Girl   *July 29, 2012*

I learned to surf today! My family is in Santa Barbara for a few days just for a little vacation and we took surfing lessons today! This is the first time that I have ever even stood on a surfboard. My mom didn't take the lessons with us but my papa, sister and I entertained her while she watched us crash, one after another in the waves! The wet suit was so uncomfortable once it got wet, it felt like it was suction cupped to my body! My dad has surfed before, in Australia, but you wouldn't know it by watching him out there. I think he fell more than I did. Anyway, after 6 hours on the water I now consider myself to be a surfer girl! By the end of the lesson we were actually getting up on the board and riding some little waves successfully. Surfing is really fun! Now I want to go again tomorrow. Santa Barbara is beautiful; I never want to leave!

The beach is my happy place, someday I am going to live near the beach where I can walk to my happy place whenever I want, breath in the ocean air, feel the sand beneath my toes and just be happy and calm. This may sound crazy, but whenever I am near the ocean I just feel better, I feel good emotionally and physically. It seems like my disease decides to go into hiding when I am near the water. Maybe my happy place really is somewhere that could be healing to me…

Chit Chat With Doctor Florida   August 1, 2012

Mommy called the doctor in Florida today. He is the same doctor who did my IgG blood tests a while back. When she called him, she explained that I am still fluctuating and that my disease flares up and down and up and down all the time! I am never at a constant. I am good for a few weeks and then it changes to bad for a few days… and then a few weeks later it changes again. This is extremely frustrating because it gets our hopes up. I can be doing awesome for weeks, normalish looking poops, no blood and no running to the bathroom. Then, in a matter of days, all of that can be back. I don't understand. One day we are celebrating a good poop and the next I am laying in bed too tired to move… And, we really do celebrate good poops. Poop is obviously not something that my family is afraid to talk about… because it has become a big part of our lives ever since I was diagnosed. This may sound bad but they actually have funny nicknames for me when I am doing well, like, "Super Pooper" or "Shitting Star" ha-ha… I love my family. We can make light of these hard situations by making up silly names like that. My family talks about poop. We talk about poop in the car, at the dinner table and while we are watching TV. "How was your poop today, Miss Heather?" Is a normal question around here.

Something I didn't really realize was that other people don't talk about poop like we do. I made a poop joke with some friends the other day and they all went "ewe that's gross" and got super uncomfortable. It wasn't even a gross joke it was about dog poop… not poop like mine… That's when I remember why I don't tell people about my disease, it would just make them uncomfortable and want to walk away and never talk to me again.

The doctor in Florida said that these fluctuations we are noticing are part of the process and not to worry about them. My colon is healing and through the healing process it will experience some bumps in the road. He told us that sometimes people get better in 6 weeks and sometimes it takes a lot longer (like years) for the gut to heal. After saying this, he then mentioned that we shouldn't add any new food challenges in to my diet for the next 6 weeks, to allow my gut to rest. Maybe we added something we shouldn't have. But what??

Few And Far Apart   *September 10, 2012*

It's been a while since I have written because everything is going pretty well. I had a great birthday last month and I am now finally 16 and driving! There are still days were I see some blood but these days are few and far apart, which I am thankful for! One thing that I have come to learn how to deal with is pain at school. Every once in a while I will just be sitting at my desk and I will feel this sharp pain in my lower left stomach. It feels like a knife stabbing into me. The pain will last for about 3 minutes and it is extremely painful. The first time that I had this pain at school I totally embarrassed myself. It came on so fast that I yelled "ouch" (out loud) and the whole class looked at me to see why I was yelling. It was such a strange pain, that I was grabbing onto my desk for dear life, and holding onto it so tight that my hands were turning white! I probably looked like an idiot but I didn't know what else to do, it came out of nowhere and hurt so bad!

Now, I am used to this pain but still handle it pretty much the same way. I grab the sides of my desk and squeeze the tabletop until the pain goes away. It is the only thing that really helps. The only thing there is to do is wait it out, but it always goes away!

Another feeling I am learning to deal with is the "poop feeling". I get this cramping feeling in my lower stomach that means 'I have to go to the bathroom NOW', but, in class I can't just run out of the room and get to the bathroom, so I have to deal with the feeling. I just lean forward and tell myself that I can't go to the bathroom right now and that I will have to wait. Now, unfortunately this doesn't always work out. There have been times where I get up to go to the bathroom like 5 times during one class period. That's when people look at me funny and wonder if I have the poops... but the funny thing is, I do!

Powder Puff!   September 17, 2012

This week is Homecoming Week and it's been a blast! Everyday is a dress up day and we come to school dressed up all funny to show our school spirit. But today is my favorite day of the spirit week, Powder Puff Football! A group of girls met up after school for practice and the football boys were our coaches. We ran drills and some of us learned how to just catch the football, because let me tell you, it is hard to grab that thing out of the air! Eventually I got it and was playing like a pro and our team was looking good. Jeff, being one of the coaches, gave me some pointers on how to take out the other team. He played catch with us and helped us warm up before the big game! My position was as a *blocker*. Basically I got to stand in front and body slam into the other girls! I really liked my position because I got to be aggressive and not have to worry about catching that crazy shaped ball. I got to run into the other girls, chase after them and take them down by grabbing their flag. I played hard. The football coach was taking pictures the whole time and he got this really great one of me in the air body slamming this girl on the other team. As aggressive as we played, we still lost. The senior team was like a bunch of men. A little beefy! There was one girl on the other team who grabbed my arms and twisted them back, and then she threw me into a puddle of mud! I was not happy about that.

Powder Puff is crazy, but fun! It's like watching a bunch of wild girls trying to attack each other, but we all look forward to this day, once a year when we get to take each other out and it's okay. Can't wait for next year! We are going to annihilate!

Volleyball From Hell — October 12, 2012

This weekend was interesting in so many ways.
We had a volleyball tournament, but it was pretty far away so they had all the teams stay in the same hotel. I was assigned to share a room with "the party girls". They brought jello shots and weed. Great. And to show their intelligence, they made the jello shots in bowls and they covered them in saran wrap and put them in their suitcases. Then when coach organized our bags in the back of the car, jello shots leaked everywhere and soaked everyone's bags. The girl whose bright idea it was to put a bowl of alcoholic jello in her duffel bag said, her "Gatorade must have spilled", and our coach bought it. I could tell this was going to be a long weekend and it was! Once we got to the hotel we were all allowed to go our separate ways for dinner. As usual, I had brought my nerdy cooler with me and was probably being made fun of but didn't care. I decided to just stick with my roommates. They chose to eat at Hooters, of course they did, and I'm stuck with them. Yippee. After spending more than enough time surrounded by half-dressed waitresses, we went back to the room. Thank goodness. But, I didn't know that meant it was time to party... and out came what was left of the jello shots. Within an hour they were all wasted and I sat there awkwardly on the couch unsure of what to do. And then, out came the weed... But, since they had nothing to smoke it out of they cut a hole in a paper cup and used that; so smart. Almost as smart as smoking pot in a hotel room and thinking that it won't stink up the place. That is when I drew the line. I got so mad at these girls because I was in the room too. First of all, I didn't want to get blamed along with all of them for the drugs and alcohol. Second, what kind of athletes are they? We had no chance of winning this tournament if everyone is hung over!

I was pissed. So I decided to go for a walk with another girl. This was a dumb idea because the girl I went with was mean and manipulative, but I guess I just wanted to get out of the room. It was like 1AM by the way. We should have been asleep! But, instead this girl took me to the pool, jumped the fence and got in. We didn't have bathing suites so we wore our sports bras and thongs, in the hot tub... horrible idea. I was so nervous the whole time that we were going to get caught!

We were fine and by the time we got back to the hotel I could smell the pot down the hallway. So, I went to get some popcorn from the front desk to mask the smell.

When I got back to the room I made the popcorn and minutes later coach knocked on our door… I opened it. She was mad that we were all still up "eating popcorn". She was pissed but didn't even notice the weed or the 6 drunk girls… I saved their butts!

The next morning was awkward because all the other girls left the door open when they went to the bathroom, but when I ran to the bathroom as soon as I woke up I wanted to close the door, clearly. The other girls made jokes about it and kept saying, "What are you doing in there?" I had half a mind to yell, "I'm shitting and it ain't pretty. Do you really wanna see?"

For obvious reasons, we got killed at the tournament and went home early. I was so annoyed. I don't like this team.

Tonight I Want To Cry   *November 11, 2012*

I don't understand. I have been crying myself to sleep. I call Jeff when I am sad and he always knows how to make me feel better. He really understands. But I don't… I am so thankful for him; he keeps my sanity. I get upset and frustrated at my disease I get angry because of how it is so unpredictable and never seems to go away, but he is always there to tell me that he loves me, sick or not and that I am strong and that we can get through this and that soon everything will be okay. He always knows exactly what to say, but I still question: *Why did this have to happen to me? Why can't I get better? I pray every night before I go to bed and I am still sick? Why?* I had a perfect poop on Monday, everything was great, and now today I feel tired and there was blood and mucus on the tissue when I wiped. I just don't get it.

I started my period yesterday and I always have some sort of emotional break down when I'm on "that time of the month", but this is different. I may be overly emotional but these are legitimate fears and reasons to be sad…

I am sad. I am sad that I get sick all the time. I am losing hope, because even when I do everything right, something goes wrong. I am scared that this will get worse and turn into colon cancer. I am angry at my disease. I am confused at why I keep getting sick. I am frustrated that nobody can figure out what is wrong with me. I just want to cry, sometimes I need to cry and just let everything out because I don't know what else to do but to just cry and scream and let all the angry out.
Tonight, I want to cry…

Spa Day

November 18, 2012

My poops are back to being good, I don't know how, the whole thing confuses me, but I'll take it!

Today was a much needed relaxation day. My mommy surprised my sister and I with a full spa day. We got facials and pedicures and massages; it was perfect. We could just relax and be pampered, this is exactly what I needed because I have been extremely stressed out about my disease lately and I know my mom needed and deserved this too. When I am scared she is scared, when I am up all night going to the bathroom, she is right there beside me. She is the one who has researched and researched and found the diet and the supplements that are keeping me out of the hospital right now. Since no medicine works and the only other option is the chemo or a drug called Lialda that all the doctors say won't work for me, we stick with the diet and the supplements. My mommy is my hero. Without her I would be lost and most likely be twice as sick. Then, they would take out my colon and give me the rest of my life to have a colostomy bag hanging from my side. My mommy and my papa have worked together to be able to find a way to save me from all of this, and they have. Merel is my best friend. She is always there to make me laugh and to be my sister. She doesn't know everything that is going on with me, because I don't want to scare her and I don't want her to think I am weak. I need to be strong for her and be there to be her big sister and her best friend. I am strong and I am not going anywhere.

We deserve this spa day.

No Chemo *December 10, 2012*

We had an appointment with the gastrointestinal specialist today. The waiting room was depressing. Today also happened to be the day that the neuro patients came in to see a different specialist because apparently he is only at this office once a week. Seeing these kids made me very anxious. Some were banging their heads against their strollers, others were shaking, some were hitting the arms of the chair and screaming, while most the rest were just sitting in their chair with their arms to their chest; they looked paralyzed. This was so sad... I couldn't handle being in there, I thought I was going to have a break down and freak out. I walked out of the waiting room and took a walk around the building to clear my head. By the time I got back it was finally my turn to see the doctor. It was about time, since we had been there for almost 2 hours...

The appointment went pretty well. I haven't had any severe diarrhea since we stopped the Asacol so it's pretty clear that Asacol is not for me... Doc said that my weight is good, blood pressure good, no fevers, and the fact that on a typical day (when I'm not in a flare) I go to the bathroom about 3 times a day is okay. Since I still have a little bleeding once in a while and I have mucus in my poop we asked if he would do another colonoscopy so that we could have an idea about what my colon looks like. I wanted to know if the mucus and blood is a warning sign or if I am healing... He didn't see a need for this and said no... he doesn't believe us that the diet is helping. He is convinced that the diet has nothing at all to do with Ulcerative Colitis and that what I eat cannot possibly affect my disease. I think that is just a stupid idea. Of course what I put through my digestive system has everything to do with the disease. It annoys me that he is so closed-minded... He won't even listen to us when we tell him that it matters. I know my body better than he does and I know that food matters. Why isn't he interested in a new finding instead of just shutting down the idea? He said I am probably just in remission and that is why the food appears to be working. He is wrong. I am learning to control my disease with the food and supplements, but he thinks I need to be on medications. What is the point of putting me on just another medication that no one can say for certain will make me better? If anything changes, he wants me on the chemo.

Is 6-MP An Option For Me?   *December 22, 2012*

So, we are at Kirkwood for a ski vacation the family, but a huge storm came in and it's been a white out for the last 2 days… there is so much snow that we can't ski. The lifts are closed. Today we tried to hike up the mountain and at least get one awesome powder run in, but ski patrol hunted us down and we got in trouble… oops!

I don't know why this time of year is so hard for me. It seems like I always get worse around Christmas. I'm not feeling so good… is it starting again? Since I am starting to flare up again we are considering the immune suppressants but won't do anything until we know exactly what we are getting into and before we know all of the risk factors. My mom did some research on the 6-MP that the doctors want me to start taking… It sounds awful. Basically it is an anti-cancer chemotherapy drug that is used to treat colitis by acting as an "Immunomodulator" which is something used to suppress immune system. So I will get the common cold or flu much easier than anyone else and it will be dangerous to me, when for everyone else it is just a cold. The medication has a slow onset – 3 to 6 months to be effective. It must be used long term. People who stop using it have bad flares. But the side effects seem the worst…they include headache, nausea, vomiting, diarrhea, and malaise (general feeling of illness) and the possibility of lupus and other diseases because of the suppressing of my immune system. When on this medication, blood tests must be performed frequently to check for negative effects on the bone marrow, liver, and kidneys.

There is no way I am taking this. It doesn't even work for everyone. If it doesn't work for me, things could be worse than they have been. Besides, so far I have been the one patient that has the impossible reactions to medications.

Super Sniffer   December 26, 2012

After doing much more research and deciding that the most recently proposed drugs do not seem like an option that I will be able to handle we found some other options. There is a lot of information about Ulcerative Colitis and only some of it is the conventional medicine idea of an autoimmune disorder. There is a doctor in New Zealand who has put together a mineral solution that is supposed to be able to kill any virus that is living in my gut. Maybe the ulcers in my colon are somehow related to the same virus that caused the shingles last year. Also, I get lots of canker sores before I get sick… We ordered these minerals after many conversations with this doctor and decided that it is worth a shot.

Today was my first day starting the minerals. There is a cycle of different minerals, all which are supposed to do a different job in cleansing my colon and killing a virus. While I am working through this protocol I will keep taking the probiotics because I have to make the good buggies happy in there and probiotics can't hurt, so what the heck. The minerals taste super salty and there is also something called "Bushlore". It's gross. The name is accurate, because its tastes like dirt and the way it works is that it comes in a little eyedropper and I have to drop 3 drops under my tongue…It is pretty icky and it smells just like it tastes… Like a bush! It's worth a try… I am open to anything right now, even some crazy minerals from a doctor in New Zealand that I have never met… I just want to be healthy again.

Speaking of smells, I have developed an amazing sniffer over the last 2 years. My family calls it the "super sniffer" because since I can't eat whatever I want, it sometimes helps satisfy my cravings if I just smell food. Like when there is a party and everyone is eating cake, I say, "Can I smell your cake?" They probably think I'm nuts, but by now, I don't care. Also, my "super sniffer" can smell every ingredient in foods! When my mommy is making dinner I can pick out everything she is using to make the meal because of my nose! Since I can't taste everything I want to, I have become way more aware of smells! My "super sniffer" can even smell things from across the room. I have a pretty obnoxious colon, but I have a pretty impressive nose to make up for it!

I Got Paid To Talk About My Poop! January 7, 2013

I actually got paid to talk about my poop. We sometimes read this blog about living with Ulcerative Colitis and there was a notice about a study recruiting kids with Ulcerative Colitis to answer a bunch of survey questions. My mom contacted the study recruiters and they actually arranged for someone to fly out from Boston, Massachusetts to interview ME.

Basically, they were designing some kind of software to survey kids about their symptoms so that doctors had a better idea of the day-to-day fluctuations that kids experience with Ulcerative Colitis. It made me sad to hear that so many kids have this terrible disease. The lady who interviewed me said that they are interviewing kids from ages 6-18. I cannot imagine this at age six! There were a lot of questions about pain, frequency of bowel movements, urgency, weight loss, fevers, sadness, etc. Right now, I am feeling really good. Based on the type of survey questions asked – I don't have it nearly as bad as some kids… But my problem has been the treatment.

It Never Ends... *January 23, 2013*

Today wasn't about me. My mom took my Papa to the emergency room. He hasn't been feeling well. Today he was all sweaty and complaining of chest pain. Turns out that he has a big blood clot in his leg and a piece of it probably broke off and went to his lungs. This is really scary, because I think this is how Uncle Marc, my papa's brother, died. Why does bad stuff keep happening to my family?

Me... I am doing fine. Ever since I started the yucky minerals and Bushlore, my poop is "normal" (it will never look like other people's poop but for having UC, this is normal). But now, there is the ACNE!! Not just a few zits. We are talking big, oozy welts on my face, my chest and my back. They are not painful like the Shingles, except for when they get touched. They aren't really zits... they are more like boils and I have no idea where they came from. Trying to explain this to my Aerobics teacher at school has not been very successful. She says, "You look fine, just do the sit-ups." I can't do sit-ups! It hurts too much to have the blisters on my back hit the floor.

Young Americans   February 7, 2013

So, this past week a traveling group of musicians, dancers and singers have come to our school to put on a big performance. A bunch of kids (including me) signed up to work with them throughout the week and we spent all week practicing for a huge musical production of singing and dancing. At the end of the week we performed and it was practically a professional performance. Our performance was last night and it was amazing! In fact, it was so incredible that we could all pass for pros! All of our hard work paid off and Jeff was right there in the audience watching me. He was so proud. My family even hosted 2 of the musicians at our house during their stay. We had 2 boys, both whom were hilarious and it was really great to have them stay with us because they worked with us individually and we learned a lot about them!

I had a blast this week and loved the performance. Young Americans was amazing!

Today I woke up with a pounding headache but otherwise everything is going great! Thank goodness! And Thank goodness I was doing well this last week, because jumping and dancing when you have irritable bowels is not fun!

Beach House! *February 16, 2013*

So, this weekend was amazing! To celebrate Valentines Day, Jeff took me to his family's beach house in Bodega Bay. We spent the weekend walking on the beach, sitting in the hot tub under the stars, playing with the puppy, watching movies, going out for romantic lunches, sight seeing and just enjoying a relaxing weekend at the beach together! It was perfect! Since I am still strictly following the diet I brought a cooler and a bag of groceries to be sure that I had food for the weekend and it worked out just fine! His mom and her friend made a delicious salmon dinner for us one night and she made sure only to use ingredients that were "Heather Safe". I am surrounded by people who really care about me and my health. Jeff and his family made going on vacation with them really easy. When we went out for meals there was always something for me and when meals were made at the house we checked all the ingredients. And, of course I brought snacks in my cooler and grocery bag so that we could nibble on "Heather Safe Snacks" throughout the day. It was a really great weekend and it was free of blood and mucus. I love the beach. The beach is my happy place and I am convinced that I feel better when I am at the beach.

Out Both Ends?! March 10, 2013

I feel like poop, which is funny because I actually haven't pooped in about 3 days. I am super constipated and I have the flu. It sucks because I feel like I have to go to the bathroom and then I will sit there for a few minutes trying to push out a log, but nothing comes out. To add to the fun I am up all night puking! I don't like it when I get sick because I always get really nervous that I am going to have a flare. It always seems to be that when I get a normal sickness that other people get all the time, I get a flare on top of it and then I just stay sick for days and it is really, well, poopy. How awful would it be to be throwing up out of one end and having bloody diarrhea out of the other end! Ewe that would be absolutely miserable!

Poopy Pants   *March 21, 2013*

My lucky duck of a sister is in Ireland right now with her violin group. I'm a wee bit jealous because I spent my few days at a children's science camp in charge of fifteen little sixth grade girls running around the cabin.

I had two special needs girls in my cabin. One had autism and did not have any friends in the cabin. The first night she sat alone on her bed, unsure of how to interact with the other girls. I noticed this and decided to play team-building games before bed. After a few games she became more comfortable around the other girls and by the end of camp, walked away with 11 new friends. I was proud to have helped this child but there was another girl I was even more thankful to have come across. The other girl wet her bed two nights in a row... It was gross but after night two, the wetting the bed turned into pooping the bed. I felt bad for her and I was sympathetic because I know the feeling... But still gross! I knew something must be wrong, because this behavior was just not normal and I remembered hearing somewhere that wetting the bed could be a sign of abuse. One morning, while in the laundry room washing her poopy pants, she confided in me. I was not expecting my suspicion of abuse to be right, so I was shocked when she said she was moved to a foster home because her father had done terrible things to her. I reported this to her teacher and the camp nurse and was assured that child welfare was aware of her case. I related to this girl in that I have pooped my pants before... but also in that we both had a challenge and she needed someone to confide in. She trusted me. Why me? Why not one of the other counselors? I think that she trusted me and knew that I would take care of her; and she was right.

We kept the whole situation a secret between us. We didn't tell other counselors and we made sure that none of the other children found out. She trusted me and I wasn't about to let her down.

This camp was also a learning experience for me with food. Clearly, I couldn't eat the corn dogs and breakfast burritos that the cook was preparing for the children. Instead, as soon as we found out that I got this job, my mommy called the camp. She talked to the cook and explained my circumstances and that I would need to bring my own food. Because of animals, I couldn't keep the food in the cabin so the cook let me keep it in the huge fridge in the kitchen. Every morning, after I got my girls all ready for the day, I would head to the kitchen and work next to the cook to make my own food. She was very understanding. I came in before every meal and prepared my own food. This worked out perfectly and I now know that I will never be held back from anything because of food. I can make my diet work wherever I am. I just have to ask for help sometimes and that is okay.

Spring Break   March 27, 2013

Over spring break my family went to Washington D.C. This is officially my new favorite city! The cherry blossoms were in bloom and the whole city was gorgeous. Now, I know they have hot summers and cold winters but the spring was beautiful! We just got back today. Over our vacation I did really well. We were able to find restaurants easy peasy and when we first got there we found a restaurant that served sourdough toast as an option for breakfast, which worked perfectly. When we go on vacation, the "bread day" thing kind of turns into a bread week… But it worked out and now that I am home I will be more careful. Overall, Washington D.C. was amazing.

The only thing I didn't get to see was the inside of the Capitol building. They have guards at the entrance of the Capitol, and one of the rules is that you can't bring food inside, and I had just bought some expensive gluten free granola that I was not about to give up. So, I hid it in my jacket…. But they found it and sent me out. I then decided I would hide my granola behind a pillar and get it when I came out. Perfect! Except for that a guard watched me hide it and when I came to the entrance she told me I was littering and could not enter the building unless I threw away the garbage I had hidden behind the pillar. Garbage, No Way! This granola was expensive and hard to find! So, partially just to spite the guards and also to save my granola I sat outside the Capitol building in the cold, and waited for my family to come out. Thankfully they weren't on a tour or anything and were only in there for about 30 minutes. Ha-ha always an adventure!

Porta-Potty

April 10, 2013

The bathrooms are locked at the tennis court and this is not okay with me. When I play tennis I run around that court and I am constantly jumping and moving around… this activates my bowels and the fact that the bathrooms are locked is not working for me.

A few days ago they brought porta-potty over to the courts. I'm not sure why they didn't just unlock the bathrooms… but now I have to use this porta-potty. My team probably wonders why I take bathroom breaks during practice. And, my poop has a tendency to smell kind nasty sometimes. Like nastier than normal poop, and it's embarrassing to stink up a porta-potty, because you can't just flush and get rid of the smell, it lingers…

Today was a weird day. I didn't feel normal but I also didn't feel sick. I just didn't feel right. There was a little bit of mucus this morning when I went potty. I finished the first phase of the Bushlore and the minerals. Now I am on another booster phase. These have the taste of licking a metal pole… We have to keep the container with the minerals in a black box in the bathroom because they are not allowed to be exposed to the sun. Three times a day I take a drink of this chemical/mineral juice. It's pretty icky. After I swallow it my face does that thing where it scrunches up, like eating something really sour. I made my whole family taste it out of solidarity and just so that they would know that the mineral water I drink 3 times a day tastes really yucky.

I am who I am   April 22, 2013

I am not a perfect person, but nobody is.
I get mad at the people who love me.
I hurt and I cry.
I laugh and I giggle; sometimes not at appropriate moments.
I may appear weak at times, but I am strong.
I smile, I cope and I keep sight of the good in the world.
I don't always know when to keep my mouth
shut or when to listen, but I try.
I don't always succeed, but I do my best.
I don't always throw myself out there, but I am outgoing.
I am always on the go, hardly resting, but I am learning.
I am always optimistic, never lost, never bored.
I seek joy in the world, but know the pain.
I am sunshine.
I create, I share and I know true happiness.
I am growing and always will be.
I will never be a perfect person, but nobody will.
I will give more than I take.
I will teach and I will learn.
I will follow my dreams and build up others.
I will never know for sure, but I will follow my heart.
I know who I am, and I believe.
I believe in smiles.
I believe in family, friends and God.
I believe each person creates their own happiness, but I believe in fate.
I believe that everything happens for a reason.

Junior Prom   *May 11, 2013*

Jeff and I are still going strong and he has been through every bump of this rollercoaster with me. Tonight was our Junior Prom. We went with two of our friends to the fanciest restaurant in town! We devoured an amazing dinner. I had filet mignon. Delicious! The best part was that someone else – I don't know who - paid for our entire meal! We didn't have to pay a penny of our tab! That is pretty awesome. I wore a beautiful salmon colored floor-length dress with my hair curled and we danced all night! It was a perfect night with the perfect guy!

Support System
May 21, 2013

Through this rollercoaster of being sick for the last 3 years and experiencing things I never thought I would have to face; I have learned the importance of a friend. Someone I trust, someone to keep my sanity, to hug me when I'm sad. Someone that I can call at 2AM crying and they will talk me through it. Someone who always knows what to say to make me feel better and someone who will drive and meet me at any time just to hold me while I cry.

For me, this person is Jeff.

Today was an extremely emotional day for me. I am frustrated. I saw blood in the toilet again today and I just broke down. I can't do this anymore! This needs to end! It is starting all over again and I can't handle it much longer... I called him crying; hysterical and scared. I told him I needed to see him and I needed him to hold me and calm me down because I don't know what to do anymore, I don't know what to tell myself or how to stop crying. I can't do this alone. He got in his car and he came and met me at the elementary school. We sat together and he held me. I told him my thoughts and my feelings and I cried and cried and cried; but that was okay, because he knows that sometimes I just need to cry. He knows that this is hard and he admires me. He knows that I am strong and he believes in me. I know he will never give up on me and he will hold my hand through anything. He told me everything would be okay and that he believes in me. He knows that this is hard and that I don't deserve this but he also knows that if anyone were strong enough to fight this battle, it is me. He told me that I can do this and that I am not alone because he is there right by my side.

This has been happening a lot lately. My mom said that people with chronic illnesses are prone to anxiety attacks and that is what this is. Mine start with a breakdown and I will curl into a ball on the floor and scream and cry and yell at the world. I freak out and seem like a crazy person, and then I cry and cry and cry. It is scary, because the only part that I can remember is crying. It is like I am not myself when I have these anxiety attacks.... It is scary, but I am lucky to have people in my life that I know are there because they want to be. They know my life is complicated but they want to be a part of it to hold my hand and help me, because they love me.

Booster Dose   June 10, 2013

I am only having a little bit of mucus and blood in the morning but that really shouldn't be the case anymore… things should be changing and even though it is just a little bit it is still scary to see in the toilet, every morning…

My mom told the doctor in New Zealand that this has been the case for a while and it isn't changing. He told us to do another booster of the minerals and the Bushlore. This means to drink MORE mineral water and MORE bush juice because maybe we didn't all the way complete phase one before we started the next cycle of chemicals, which is just as gross as the first. They taste the same but apparently they are different. We don't know what to do anymore. I am afraid to continue with a treatment that nobody here seems to know about or understand.

Once A Counselor, Always A Counselor   July 18, 2013

Just like last summer I am working at the children's summer camp! I really love working with children and actually enjoy my job. I get paid to play with kids all day; it's great!

These kids love me and they really trust me. They always want to be holding my hand or grabbing onto my leg, but sometimes I want them to leave me alone... like, for example, when I go to the bathroom... I don't especially want six little five year olds huddled around the bathroom stall waiting for me to finish and come out... why? Well, because sometimes my poop sounds a little more explosive than others, and even though they are six, its still embarrassing. They are six but they still know that poop shouldn't sound like a cannon, and if they hear that mine does, there will be lots of awkward questions that I don't want to answer.
I love them, but I don't want them in the bathroom.

My Birthday Is Jinxed

August 27, 2013

I swear my birthday must be jinxed. Every year something seems to happen… This year, there is a huge fire destroying miles and miles of forest where we live and we have been evacuated. To get out of the smoke we decided to make the best of the situation and head to the beach to celebrate my birthday. I love being near the ocean.

One In A Million
September 3, 2013

My mom and I saw this cool test online that anyone can do, at home, to see if you have a systemic yeast infection! We thought, what the heck, maybe I have yeast or even parasites?! It's a spit test, and we have been noticing that my spit is really thick and stringy, unlike other peoples…SO, we did the test. It was actually really cool. The way it worked is that we fill up our own cup with water and first thing in the morning, we spit in our cups. We all did it, my mom, my papa, my sister and me. Then we watched our spit wad change. Mine, turned into strings reaching from top to bottom and almost looked like a spider web in the glass. My mom's just floated like normal spit would do, then kind of dissolved - Same for my dad and sister. Hmm…based on that little at-home test, I have systemic yeast, maybe even parasites! Yay… maybe I should get tested for real. We haven't even considered parasites for while, but we know my body has some bad bugs.

So, my mom contacted these specialists at a digestive health center in New York. They said they have worked with lots of people with Ulcerative Colitis and yeast problems. My mommy had a long phone consult with this new doctor in New York who specializes in using herbal remedies to "cure" Ulcerative Colitis. He said he would work with us… so, once again, why not? It's worth a shot. I mean, what else are we going to do, we are pretty much out of options and I am still not ready to accept a life of being on drugs that suppress my immune system, and surgery is not even a consideration. So, more herbs and supplements.

Bad Night With The Herbs   September 12, 2013

Something bad happened. The herbs and oils are not really working out so great. I started introducing these strange oils; like peppermint oil, oregano oil, black walnut oil…. Anyway, things didn't go so well with the oils. The doctor told us to start slowly and to rotate them every fourth day and they would help kill the bacteria. This is exactly what we did, but it didn't help kill the bacteria, or maybe it did but it tried to kill me in the process. I was actually choking on mucus AND having diarrhea all night long. Like my body just had to get rid of all of these things. Like I had said, it was the worst thing ever… I was puking while having diarrhea! I actually had to hold a bucket on my lap while I sat on the toilet… It was so gross. It was exactly the same result as I had with the Ciprofloxacin two years ago! Diarrhea and Blood and Mucus! Yuck… most teenage girls squeal at the sight of a paper cut, but me, I'm have gotten used to blood.

My mom called the doctor… again. Apparently this had never happened to anyone before. He didn't know what to tell us, because this wasn't supposed to happen… Here I am, once again that one-in-a-million person that nobody can figure out. One more time, the impossible seems to be possible with me. Why can't I just be normal!? So, the plan is to change the herbs and supplements. Who ever knew that herbs could be so potent! I was actually doing o.k. - not great but o.k. The promise of a "cure" seemed worth a try, but not now.

Stress

October 20, 2013

I can't even remember the last time that I have gone to sleep without actually crying myself to sleep. This has all become too much for me. The constant trial and what seems to be the never-ending failure. I freak out at my family a lot! I usually don't even remember what freaks me out. I can't concentrate at school, I have cramps all the time, I am angry, I am sad and it seems like the only thing to do is scream at my family.

I met my Jeff at the elementary school again yesterday. I feel bad. I feel like I am a burden to him and an extra stressor that he doesn't need. As hard as this journey has been for me, I know it has been hard for all those close to me as well. I don't want to push him away with all my craziness. I need him. I need him to be there to hold me and to calm me down. I am scared about my disease and how lost and confused everyone is in trying to treat it. I am worried that I will never be healthy again. Scared I will never see a normal healthy poop in the toilet. To add to my worries, I am scared for my dad, his health and his condition. I am scared that because my dad's disease is genetic that I will have that illness to add to my list. I am scared and this is all too much for me to handle alone. I am just a kid.

Even though it is a big responsibility for such young people to have to handle, I am thankful that I have my boyfriend here to help me through all of this. I know that this is hard on him too and sometimes I think I shouldn't share all of this with him because I don't want to stress him out. But when I asked him if I should stop telling him things, he said, *"No, I want to be here for you and I don't want you to ever feel like you can't talk to me."* Well, that solves that problem. I don't have to worry about stressing him out anymore. Phewwy! That's one thing I can cross off my list!

I know that stress is bad and that it makes my disease flare, but really, try being in this situation or any situation that stress could affect and try not to stress…. It's impossible!

Now I'm "Poopy Pants" October 29, 2013

I pooped my pants. I actually pooped my pants. And, that isn't even the best part.... I pooped my pants, at school. Now, what is more embarrassing than that? Pooping your pants, at school, when your 17! Yeah, not much comes to mind.

So, the story goes like this:

I was in my Theory of Sports class just minding my own business, taking notes and I get "the feeling". I know that I need to go to the bathroom NOW but I am worried that if I stand up I will "let it out." I tried to hold it in, but that didn't work. I needed to go NOW. I got up and ran. I RAN out of the classroom. Everyone saw. No bathroom pass or anything, I didn't even ask the teacher if I could go. I just ran. But, I still didn't make it. About half way to the bathroom I knew it was coming out. I couldn't make it. There was no way. Then, I squatted. Right there in the middle of my High School campus, I squatted and I shit my pants. Just like that. Then... I had to walk to the bathroom, with a load in my pants. Now, the best part is these pants weren't just jeans or something that the poop wouldn't be terribly noticeable in... No; I was wearing light grey yoga pants. It was awful. You could see everything, straight through; mushy brown poop filled with mucus and blood. It's disgusting. I get to the bathroom and thankfully I'm the only one in there. I locked the door and took my pants off, cleaned them in the sink and dried them under the hand drier. Tied my sweatshirt around my waist. Good as new. But still...Ewe. Crying at how embarrassed and sad I am; I am still trying to digest the fact that I just pooped my pants at school. I called my Jeff. He is out of town with a friend. At a time like this when I really need him, he just has to be out of town... His week away hasn't even started and I can't go a day without him before I start pooping my pants, literally... The first thing I said to him was "I had an accident at school" and he answered, "Did you make it?"... "No, I pooped my pants..." He told me to call my mommy and to just go home. That's exactly what I did. This is going to be a long week.

We are stopping this herbal supplement thing... It is just making everything worse.

Shit!
November 6, 2013

Last night, after my shift volunteering in the emergency room my mommy met me for dinner. I felt better today so we went out to our favorite restaurant. I ordered fries and a steak. Probably the wrong choice since it might be a bit heavy on the digestion. But I was so hungry! We had eaten there before with no problems. I felt fine at dinner and we had a nice evening. Then when we went to our separate cars to drive home, things started to go south for me.

I was driving along, happy as could be, rocking out to Keith Urban when I got "the feeling" again. It was coming on fast and I didn't know what to do… I can't poop in my car. So, I pulled over quickly, left the car running, ran around the side and exploded all over the side of the road. I felt so bad because I went right by someone's mailbox… and this could not have passed as a doggie doo-doo. Thankfully my friend and I had been out TP-ing her boyfriend's house a few nights before so I had toilet paper in my car. (I think I am going to leave that roll in my car for a while, it seems to be something that comes in handy lately) I covered up my mess and tried to scoot it away from the mailbox. It isn't exactly solid, so that was difficult. This pooping my pants thing is gross. Everyone has probably had the experience of having to pee so bad they stop the car and go on the side of the road. I'm sure lots of people have even had to stop the car to throw up on the side of the road. But to poop? That is so embarrassing. What kind of 17 year old girl shits herself? That isn't lady like at all!

Run Run Run To The Bathroom November 11, 2013

I have aerobics first period. And, little bowel fact: the bowel is most active in the morning. That is why most people poop when they wake up, like me! And another bowel fact: running makes your bowels more active! So… if you put two and two together it would make sense that running in the morning isn't so fun for people with Ulcerative Colitis. At least not when they are in a flare like I am…

I go the most in the morning. So, since running in the morning sounds awful it makes it fantastic that I have aerobics first period and have to run at least a mile every class day… I can't do it. I literally start running, get the feeling, change course and head straight to the bathroom! Yay for me. The whole class probably thinks I get the shits really easy and the funny thing is that they are spot on! I don't think I am going to be able to stay in this class first period if every time I run, I have to poop…. Not to mention jumping jacks and sit ups. Those don't help the situation much either.

My mom is freaking out! I don't blame her. I am a mess that nobody can seem to clean up. She called her close friend who works as a nurse with a GI Doctor in town. She told her my story and vented her frustrations… Her friend mentioned that the doctor she works with is really great and that we should try to work with him. We definitely need someone to help us. The New York guy took me off all the supplements and suggested we start the "Specific Carbohydrate Diet." I hate this so much. What I don't get is why one set of doctors recommends I take drugs to suppress my immune system and another group of doctors recommends that I change the way I eat. None of this makes any sense.

Thanksgiving On The SCD
November 27, 2013

So we started the Specific Carbohydrate Diet a few weeks ago and I immediately began to feel better. The bleeding and diarrhea stopped. I hate not having any bread, potatoes, rice, fruits… but what is the alternative? My mom brought cookbooks and cooked all of the food for me at my Aunt's house in Colorado. The "Heather Safe Foods" had little stickers on the bowls. Everyone shared and said they like my food. Yeah, well nobody understands that I HAVE to eat like this. I miss just eating food like a normal person. My mom even packed a yogurt maker. Who takes a yogurt maker on vacation?

Food DOES Matter — December 14, 2013

So we did the Specific Carbohydrate Diet for a few weeks and that went surprisingly, horrible! It worked for about 2 weeks and then, didn't work. On that diet I couldn't eat any rice, potatoes, wheat or anything with sugar, so I am slightly happy that it didn't work out, because I don't think I could go the rest of my life without carbs or sugar! Apparently, I was eating something that my body could not handle. Now we are back to the low salicylate diet. At least the list of foods includes things I like, AND I am feeling good. I can still feel that things are not normal but I am so much better than I was a few weeks ago. The urgency is gone, the bleeding is almost completely gone and the pain is under control. Once again, for me the impossible seems possible.

Doctor Number 8   December 18, 2013

We took my mom's friend's advice and called the doctor, but, he is an adult doctor and I am 17… Mom's friend explained my situation to the doctor and he decided I was close enough to 18 and physically in an adult body so he would make room for me on his patient list. I am super nervous to meet this guy; doctors haven't worked out so well for me… hopefully this one will. My mom and her friend came to school to get me; we were all going to this appointment together. Since I have gone through so many doctors and all of them have been a bust, my mom was just as nervous as I was. So, she brought her friend along for support. I was freaking out inside. Doctors are scary!

Since I went back to the low salicylate diet a few days ago I have been feeling a lot better. When we looked back at my medical history that was the diet that I was doing the best on. We know that food is a factor we just aren't completely sure which foods yet. Also, we stopped all the supplements except the probiotics. It almost seems impossible that I have been doing so much better the last week! It's crazy how fast my colon can change.

This new doctor came across as a jerk at first. He said he didn't believe that food mattered, but I know that it does. Then, after about an hour-long appointment, he opened his mind to the idea and understands my situation more. He realized that we have been following professional advice and doing what we are told, but nothing seems to have been a lasting solution. He wants to work with me and he wants to help us find a way to treat this incurable monster. But, first he has to know what's going on. He wants to take a peek… You know what that means? Colonoscopy time!

Happy Holidays!   *December 23, 2013*

Today was colonoscopy day! Two days before Christmas I get an itty-bitty camera stuck up my butt. The results did not come out as well as we hoped they would. Actually the results were pretty bad... At my last colonoscopy I only had a little bit of inflammation at the very end of my colon. Today we found out that the entire length of my colon is now inflamed.

I have two options:

1.) Chemo/6-MP medication that has a long list of extreme side effects
2.) A different type of mesalamine drug called Lialda

Chemo is really a last resort for us, because I think the chances of me getting worse or developing other diseases are way too high! The option of Lialda was brought up before at many doctors' appointments in the past but we were always told it wasn't an option for me. The previous doctors told us that Lialda was just an expensive drug that is exactly like the Asacol; This doctor disagrees. He says we need to do something because I cannot go without treating this much inflammation. We came to a conclusion: We are going to try the Lialda and I will be on Prednisone for three months as well to help bring all the inflammation down. That means puffy cheeks, fat tummy and zits... gross, but better than bloody poop. Also, I am going to stay on the low salicylate diet. Here we go again; worth a shot.

All Good Things Take Time *January 15, 2014*

Right now I am taking VSL3 probiotics, vitamin B (for my emotions and stress), Lialda and the prednisone. I am also still following the dietary restriction- these aren't as hard as previous diets because I get to eat ice cream and bread once in a while. Things are going great! No blood. No mucus. No diarrhea. I haven't felt this good in over three years; it's a wonderful feeling!

Of course…I do have to remember that I am on a pretty high doses of steroids (prednisone) right now, so I can't really know for sure if it's the Lialda that is working because it could just be the prednisone that is working or it could be the diet. We don't really know. Time will tell, but for right now, life is back to the way it was before. Well, except for the handful of pills and the diet; but I am healthy again. My prayers have been answered. It took about 4 years, but hey, all good things take time.

The Drive To Keep Going   March 22, 2014

I haven't been writing much because there is nothing to say. Life is wonderful! I am strong, healthy and I have seen a formed poop in the toilet for the last 2 and a half months. It's a miracle. We are tapering off the prednisone now (no more puffiness) and things seem to be working. The Lialda is not making me sick like the other medications did. Those doctors who always told me that Lialda wasn't an option were wrong. I wish we had found out about this medication years ago, but then again, I am thankful for this journey I have been on. Through it I have found endless support, strength, resilience, hope and the drive to keep pushing through. I know that this medication works for me, but it isn't a cure. It simply covers up the side effects and brings down the inflammation in my colon; but I still have Ulcerative Colitis. My doctor has now started listening to me about my background with food and realizes that food truly does matter. We have agreed that for now I should continue the dietary restrictions and then gradually, overtime I can add back more foods. Eventually, we are hoping that there will only be two or three foods that I react to. For now, I am right where I want to be. Life is good and I finally found a doctor that will listen to me.

It's Time To Say Goodbye   March 27, 2014

It is time to stop writing in this journal. I am healthy, happy and strong; the only things that I have longed for over the most difficult last 4 years of my life, and now I have those things. I am back. Healthy, Happy Heather is back and she is here to stay. I have overcome my battle. Although, my story is not over and neither is my journey, I feel that my struggle has come to an end.

I have found a balance between diet and medication and I know that is what works for me. My treatment has been difficult to resolve but all of the trial and error was worth it. Without all of the hard times and the defeat, I would not have been able to find what works for me.

I am going to be Okay. I no longer have to worry. I am leaving for college in the fall on a campus near the ocean and I feel ready to manage this on my own. I will be in my happy place and I am ready for the next chapter in my story and look forward for what life has to offer.

In one month I will be running a half marathon and I fully intend to run the whole thing. I am strong enough now. I know that I will run all 13.1 miles and pass every porta potty along the way, without stopping. I don't have to worry about that anymore.

I will continue to travel and to see the world and I hope to go on to med-school where I can become the doctor that I had such a hard time finding. A doctor that will understand not only one's illness but also what it is like to be chronically ill and understand that it's scary. But I'm not scared anymore.

I hope that my story can help others to find their inner strength and resilience; their drive to keep going even when life is so hard that they don't want to keep fighting anymore. I don't want others to give up. Fight! Because even though the journey is hard and may take years, the last person you want to give up on in life is yourself.

Anything is possible.

Every time doctors told me something was Impossible, I learned to believe that *I'm*possible.

Appendix (and Colon ☺ *)*

I have been blessed with a burden.

I have come to think part of life is learning to handle the burdens that are thrown at us. Everyone has their own burden to carry and no one burden is greater than another. The difference from one's burden and another's is how they choose to handle it. Everyone knows that person who goes around complaining about how their life is so hard. I was never that person. I was the person people looked at and said, "Man I wish I had a life as easy as hers", because nobody knew about my burdens and my fears. I kept smiling and I didn't feel I needed to advertise my struggles. I was happy and that's all people needed to know. I had the people in my life who were there for me, and who I could lean on when times got hard; but as for everybody else, why do they need to know?

Sometimes I feel frustrated hearing people talk about how hard their life is and how they just can't handle it anymore. Over the past few years I have listened to classmates who complain of "stomach problems" but they eat junk, drink alcohol and don't do anything to keep their body healthy. I sat quietly and listened while other kids complained and looked around the room at the silent kids, wondering what they had to say. Sometimes the biggest story comes from the one with the least to say.

Everyone carries a weight on their shoulders. Many times I had to bite my lip when I heard kids complain and make up diseases or when other kids had been drunk all weekend or were on drugs. Maybe that is their coping mechanism. They just don't understand. The same way I wouldn't understand what it is like to have divorced parents or a father in jail. I have come to know how important it is to take care of your body. It hurt me to meet children who had been hurt by others at such a young age. Just as it hurt to have my life change without me being ready to face my new struggles. Having to reassess my world one day and decide that I was going to make it work, was hard. But watching other people throw their life away when I know they have so much to offer, is painful. I learned all of this at a young age because life brought me my challenges at that age. Not only did I spend high-school studying and making friends but I spent it battling the most difficult 4 years of my life and learning that life is precious and is meant to be cherished.

Favorite Recipes:

Since I don't eat eggs anymore, we substitute homemade yogurt with a little bit of baking soda for the eggs. I try not to eat a lot of wheat/gluten, so we go gluten-free most of the time. Except for sourdough bread. I love toasted sourdough bread with butter!

Homemade Yogurt: (we use the *Yo'gourmet* electric yogurt maker.) Learning to make our own yogurt has been fun and allows yogurt to be used in lots of recipes. Yummy, with lots of good bugs for my tummy.

Ingredients:

> 1 gallon of whole milk (we use organic)
> Two 5 gram packages of Freeze dried yogurt starter by *Yo'gourmet*.

Using a clean pan, bring the milk to a gentle boil. Go slowly, stir frequently and be careful not to let it burn.

Allow milk to cool to room temperature.

Prepare yogurt maker by plugging in and adding warm water to the level indicated.

Add one cup of the cooled milk and the two 5 gram packages of yogurt starter to the inner container of the yogurt maker. Still well.

Add remaining milk to the inner container of the yogurt maker.

Let cook in yogurt maker for at least 24 hours, but not longer than 30 hours.

Refrigerate inner container and enjoy!

Gluten Free Oatmeal Cookies:

Ingredients:

    6 Tablespoons of butter softened to room temperature
    ½ cup of white sugar
    ½ cup of brown sugar
    3 eggs – *we substitute 3 large tablespoons of homemade yogurt*
    1 ½ cup of gluten free oatmeal flakes
    ½ cup of sweet sorghum flour
    ½ tsp of baking soda
    ½ tsp of baking powder – *we use the one with potato starch not corn*
    ¼ tsp salt
    Chocolate chips – *we use the EnJoy Life brand*

Preheat oven to 350 degrees.
Using electric mixer, blend butter and sugars together until smooth.
Blend in the sweet sorghum flour and salt until mixture is smooth and moist.
By hand, stir in the yogurt, oatmeal flakes, baking soda and baking powder. Let mixture sit for a few minutes after stirring all together. (This allows the oatmeal to soak up the moisture.)
By hand, stir in about ½ cup of chocolate chips. More or less as you like.

Place small balls of dough onto baking sheet and bake 10-12 minutes. Let cool before removing from pan. This is tricky! If you remove them too soon, they break, if you wait too long, they stick.

If too greasy, you can add a bit more sorghum flour. For a fun variation, add about ¼ cup of ground cashew flour. Enjoy!

Cream of Asparagus Soup:

We make our own chicken stock by boiling chicken bones in water with fresh garlic and fresh celery. This stock can then be used to make a variety of different soups. This is one of my favorites!

Ingredients:

- 1 pound of asparagus
- 1 large yellow onion
- 3 tablespoons butter
- 4 cups homemade chicken stock
- 1 cup of water
- 2 tablespoons fresh chopped parsley
- ¼ cup heavy cream
- a squeeze of fresh lemon juice
- salt to taste

Cut the woody stems and the tips of asparagus off. Discard the stems and save the tips for garnish. Chop the remaining asparagus into small rounds.

Chop the onion into small pieces.

Melt the butter into a large pan and then add asparagus and onion, cooking until onions become translucent – about 5 minutes. Sprinkle with salt while cooking.

Add the chicken stock and water, bringing to a soft boil. Lower heat and continue cooking for approx. 15 minutes until asparagus is tender.

Remove from heat, add chopped parsley and let cool.

Blend in food processor until smooth. Add cream and a bit of fresh lemon juice. Warm to serve. Enjoy!

Pizza:

Everyone loves pizza! My mom figured out how to make "Heather Safe" pizza.

Crust Ingredients:

> 1 ½ cups brown rice flour
> ½ cup potato flour
> 1 tablespoon tapioca flour
> 1 tablespoon yeast
> 1 tablespoon sugar
> ¼ cup homemade yogurt
> 2 tablespoons canola oil
> warm water
> Salt

Topping Ingredients:

> Fresh tomato
> Garlic
> Fresh grated parmesan cheese
> Prosciutto
> Sweet yellow onion
> Fresh grated white cheddar cheese / goat cheese

Set oven to 425 degrees.

CRUST:
Add the yeast and sugar to ½ cup of warm water, allowing 10 minutes for yeast to multiply.

Mix all other dry ingredients together and then stir in yogurt and canola oil.

Add yeast mixture to other ingredients, stirring by hand and slowly adding warm water until dough reaches a moist, sticky texture. Salt to taste.

Cover and let rise for 20-30 minutes while preparing the toppings.

Form dough to pizza pan and cook for approx. 6 minutes before adding toppings.

TOPPINGS:

Plunge whole tomato into boiling water for a few minutes. Rinse until cool and then remove the skin. Cut in half and remove seeds.

Place peeled tomato in blender with 2 cloves of garlic and approx. ¼ cup grated parmesan cheese.

Spread tomato mixture over pre-baked crust. Add prosciutto, onion, and grated white cheese.

Bake additional 12-16 minutes. Enjoy!

Made in the USA
Middletown, DE
25 April 2021